A Comprehensive Text Book on Self-emulsifying Drug Delivery Systems

Edited by

Deepak Kaushik

&

Ravinder Verma

Department of Pharmaceutical Sciences
Maharshi Dayanand University, Rohtak
India

A Comprehensive Text Book on Self-emulsifying Drug Delivery Systems

Editor: Deepak Kaushik and Ravinder Verma

ISBN (Online): 978-981-4998-00-0

ISBN (Print): 978-981-4998-01-7

ISBN (Paperback): 978-981-4998-02-4

©2021, Bentham eBooks imprint.

Published by Bentham Science Publishers Pte. Ltd. Singapore. All Rights Reserved.

BENTHAM SCIENCE PUBLISHERS LTD.
End User License Agreement (for non-institutional, personal use)

need for a court order if at any point you breach any terms of this License Agreement. In no event will any delay or failure by Bentham Science Publishers in enforcing your compliance with this License Agreement constitute a waiver of any of its rights.

3. You acknowledge that you have read this License Agreement, and agree to be bound by its terms and conditions. To the extent that any other terms and conditions presented on any website of Bentham Science Publishers conflict with, or are inconsistent with, the terms and conditions set out in this License Agreement, you acknowledge that the terms and conditions set out in this License Agreement shall prevail.

Bentham Science Publishers Pte. Ltd.
80 Robinson Road #02-00
Singapore 068898
Singapore
Email: subscriptions@benthamscience.net

BENTHAM SCIENCE

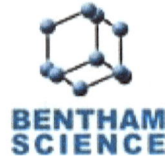

CONTENTS

FOREWORD

Self-emulsifying drug delivery system (SEDDS) is a significant approach for improving the rate and extent of absorption of hydrophobic or lipophilic drugs that come under class II and IV of the Biopharmaceutical Classification System (with low solubility), and exhibits a dissolution rate-limited absorption. SEDDS formulations lead to increased drug solubility and bioavailability, avoidance of food effect, and enhanced environmental degradation stability. Enhanced oral bioavailability allows dose reductions and high efficiency of drug release. In the gastrointestinal tract (GIT), self-emulsifying formulations spread readily, and the digestive motility of the stomach and intestine provides the stimulation required for self-emulsification.

This reference book on SEDDS specifically addresses the basic aspects and current research going on in this field. In the following nine chapters, various authors give a comprehensive review of SEDDS, covering the basic components and latest advances such as solid-SMEDDS, herbal SEDDS formulations along with discussions on pharmacokinetic and *in vitro* digestion models for estimation of SEDDS.

The book is an excellent reference work for academicians, students, pharmaceutical industry professionals as well as research scientists involved in the investigation and development of SEDDS.

Arun Nanda
Department of Pharmaceutical Science
M.D.University, Rohtak
India

PREFACE

The book "A Comprehensive textbook on self-emulsifying drug delivery systems" will cater to both pharmaceutical academics and industry professionals involved in the area of Formulation, Development and Research. The book presents a complete insight on self-emulsifying formulations providing an in-depth understanding of the basic aspects and mechanisms of these formulations and details about the current research and development in this field. This book is specially meant for research students and other professionals who carry out their research in the field of development of Lipid-Based Drug Delivery Systems, especially Self-Micro Emulsifying Drug Delivery Systems for the oral dosage form.

The major contents of the current book are the following:

- The first chapter is introductory where various techniques of oral bioavailability enhancement such as size reduction, crystal habit modification, complexation, inclusion complex, solubilization with co-solvents or surfactants, drug dispersion with carriers (*e.g.* eutectic mixture, solid dispersion and polymeric carriers) like micro/nanoemulsions, self-emulsifying drug delivery systems, liposomes, solid lipid nanoparticles, nanostructured lipid carriers and so on are discussed briefly.
- The second chapter reviews various lipid-based drug delivery systems such as emulsion, microemulsion, nanoemulsion, liposomes, solid lipid nanoparticles, self-emulsifying drug delivery systems, self-microemulsifying drug delivery systems, self-nanoemulsifying drug delivery system and so on which are summarized with their pros and cons.
- The third chapter describes the self micro-emulsifying drug delivery systems (SMEDDS) and their applications in various fields such as pharmaceutical (self-microemulsion, cosmetics agents), chemical (analytical purpose, enzymatic reactions, immobilization of protein) and industrial processes (bioseparations by microemulsion, chemical sensor materials).
- The fourth chapter provides an insight into various components of self-emulsifying formulations such as lipids, surfactants and co-surfactants. The fifth chapter provides a discussion on the mechanism and aspects of lymphatic transportation of self-emulsifying formulations. The factors affecting the lymphatic transport of these formulations are also highlighted. Theco-surfactants are major components of these formulations and are described in detail alongwith their functions and appropriate examples. These components are meant for achieving maximum drug loading, minimal self-emulsification time and droplet size in the gastric environment for obtaining maximum assimilation, to lessen the variation in the emulsion globule size and to prevent or minimize drug degradation/precipitation.
- The sixth chapter explains the advantages, drawbacks and evaluation parameters of self-emulsifying formulations along with a brief discussion on marketed self-emulsifying formulations.
- The seventh chapter is focused on Solid-SMEDDS which represents solid dosage formulation with self-emulsification features. Various solidification strategies and types of solid SMEDDS are discussed briefly along with their benefits and drawbacks.
- The eighth chapter provides a discussion on a variety of herbal drugs and conventional pharmaceuticals being exploited for the formulation of SMEDDS. The herbal self-emulsifying formulations containing extracts or volatile and fixed oils such as zedoary

turmeric oil, quercetin, silymarin, baicalein, hesperidin, gentiopicrin and so on are summarized in this chapter.
• The ninth chapter explains the pharmacokinetics parameters and *in vitro* digestion models along with relevant examples for estimation of SMEDDS.

The editors sincerely thank all the authors who have contributed to the successful completion of this book. We would like to thank Bentham Science Publishers for their support and efforts in reaching this book in its final shape.

Deepak Kaushik

&

Ravinder Verma
Department of Pharmaceutical Science
M.D.University, Rohtak
India

List of Contributors

Anurag Khatkar   Department of Pharmaceutical Sciences, Maharshi Dayanand University, Rohtak (Haryana), 124001, India

Beena Kumari   Department of Pharmaceutical Sciences, Indra Gandhi University, Meerpur, Rewari, India

Deepak Kaushik   Department of Pharmaceutical Sciences, Maharshi Dayanand University, Rohtak (Haryana), 124001, India

Deepak Parmar   Department of Chemistry, Maharshi Dayanand University, Rohtak (Haryana), 124001, India

Deepika Purohit   Department of Pharmaceutical Sciences, Indra Gandhi University, Meerpur, Rewari, India

Manish Kumar   M.M. College of Pharmacy, Mullana, Ambala, Haryana, India

Pawan Jalwal   Shri Baba Mastnath Institute of Pharmaceutical Sciences and Research, Baba Mastnath University, Rohtak (Haryana), 124001, India

Prerna Kaushik   Department of Pharmaceutical Sciences, Maharshi Dayanand University, Rohtak (Haryana), 124001, India

Parijat Pandey   Shri Baba Mastnath Institute of Pharmaceutical Sciences and Research, Baba Mastnath University, Rohtak (Haryana), 124001, India

Ravinder Verma   Department of Pharmaceutical Sciences, Maharshi Dayanand University, Rohtak (Haryana), 124001, India

Rekha Rao   Department of Pharmaceutical Sciences, Guru Jambheshwar University, Hisar (Haryana), India

Ritu Kaushik   Department of Pharmaceutical Sciences, Maharshi Dayanand University, Rohtak (Haryana), 124001, India

Sarita Khatkar   Vaish Institute of Pharmaceutical Education and Research, Rohtak (Haryana), 124001, India

Vineet Mittal   Department of Pharmaceutical Sciences, Maharshi Dayanand University, Rohtak (Haryana) 124001, India

Vandana Singh   Department of Pharmaceutical Sciences, Maharshi Dayanand University, Rohtak (Haryana), 124001, India

CHAPTER 1

Different Methodologies for Improving Solubility and Bioavailability

Ravinder Verma[1], Deepak Kaushik[1,*], Ritu Kaushik[1] and **Vandana Singh[1]**

[1] *Department of Pharmaceutical Sciences, Maharshi Dayanand University, Rohtak (Haryana), 124001, India*

Abstract: Drug delivery through the oral route is perfect for both solid and liquid dosage forms. Notwithstanding numerous favorable circumstances, the improvement of the oral delivery route still speaks to an excellent test attributable to interesting curious physicochemical characteristics of lipophilic drug compounds and physiological barriers, such as gastrointestinal unsteadiness, pre-systemic metabolism and efflux pump. Upon oral intake, lipophilic drug in a dosage form is effortlessly taken by patients, passes the GIT *via* a tremendously versatile environment. Factors affecting solubilization are the size of particle, temperature, pressure, molecular size, nature of solute and solvent, polarity and polymorphs. Ways of enhancing oral bioavailability includeboth chemical modifications and formulation modifications. The chemical modification includes soluble pro-drug and salt formation. While formulation modification comprises of physical changes like size reduction, crystal habit modification, complexation (*e.g.* with β-cyclodextrin), solubilization with co-solvents or surfactants, drug dispersion with carriers (*e.g.* eutectic mixture, solid dispersion and polymeric carriers like micro/nanoemulsions, self-emulsifying drug delivery systems, liposomes, solid lipid nanoparticles (SLNs) and nanostructured lipid carriers which are described briefly. A formulation approach is a preferable option to chemical modification approaches which may prompt the change in chemical structure and may have an impact on the pharmacological action. Particle size reduction is classified into two categories - mechanical micronization and engineered particle size control. Mechanical micronization includes jet milling, ball milling, high-pressure homogenization. Engineered particle size control includes the cryogenic method, spray freezing onto cryogenic fluids, spray freezing into cryogenic liquids, spray freezing into vapor over liquid, ultra-rapid freezing and cryogenic spray processes. Crystal engineering includes nanocrystals, solid dispersion, co-crystal formation, sonocrystallization, liquisolid technique, self-microemulsifying drug delivery systems and inclusion complex which are discussed in detail. This chapter highlights various methods for solubility enhancements with their merits and demerits.

Keywords: Crystal engineering, Cryogenic method, High-pressure homogenization, Liposomes, Nanostructured lipid carriers, Oral bioavailability.

---

* **Corresponding author Deepak Kaushik:** Department of Pharmaceutical Sciences, Maharshi Dayanand University, Rohtak (Haryana), 124001, India; Tel: +91 9315809626; E-mail: deepakkaushik1977@gmail.com

INTRODUCTION

The oral route is the most favorable route for the administration of the drug owing to its multiple benefits such as ease of administration, strong patient compliance, possibility of different release options, cost-effectiveness, self-administration, convenience for prolonged repeated use, the most valuable non-invasive and the most common route for the treatment of various diseases.

Drug delivery through the oral route is perfect for both solid and liquid dosage forms. Liquid dosage forms are noticeable because of the simplicity of administration, the precision of measurements, self-administration, pain avoidance and especially patient compliance [1].

As our human body comprises around 70% water, a drug must be soluble in aqueous GIT fluid to have adequate bioavailability. The drug present in the dosage forms discharges in gastrointestinal (GI) fluid after its breaks down that results in a solution after gentle agitation. This process is solubility dependent. The passage of the solution form of a drug across the cell lining membrane in the GI tract is permeability constrained. Then, the drug assimilates into the blood. The oral bioavailability of a drug is measured by the rate of drug solubility and permeability.

DIFFICULTIES IN THE ORAL DRUG DELIVERY

Notwithstanding numerous favorable circumstances, the oral drug delivery is a big challenge due to complex physicochemical characteristics of lipophilic drug compounds and physiological conditions. Gastrointestinal contents, pre-systemic metabolism, aqueous solubility, drug permeability, drug extent of dissolution and efflux pumps are some of the complex factors which affect the efficiency of drug administration through the oral route. Oral intake of lipophilic drug in a dosage form is effortlessly taken by patients, goes in GIT *via* a tremendously versatile environment. When a drug transits from a highly acidic pH to the digestive system, the stomach digestive enzymes and microflora alter its pH. In this perspective, the main issues of oral delivery are the physicochemical characteristics of drugs and physiological conditions of human body [2].

ORAL BIOAVAILABILITY

The majority of the new chemical compounds being worked on nowadays are planned to be utilized as solid dosage forms so that a viable and reproducible *in vivo* plasma concentration can be acquired after oral administration. In any case, poor retention and poor bioavailability do not allow oral route for intake of numerous drugs. That is why in many cases, injections are preferred for administration of such therapeutic moieties, for example, proteins and peptides due to their poor oral bioavailability that prompts high fluctuation and poor control of plasma concentrations and therapeutic effects.

The process of drug dissolution is vital for the therapeutic efficacy of the orally administered drug and route of intake. Drug dissolution includes the transfer of a solid drug into the aqueous phase in the physiological fluid. The dissolution extent of a drug is influenced by factors incorporated in the Noyes-Whitney equation [3].

REASON FOR POOR ORAL BIOAVAILABILITY

Less bioavailability is frequently connected with the drugs related to BCS II, III and IV. Drugs such as acyclovir, aspirin, atorvastatin, simvastatin, ibuprofen *etc.* with less water solubility and less permeability or both as are shown in Fig. (**1**).

There are a few reasons which are credited for poor bioavailability of drug. These components include drug properties, dosage form, solubility, acid-base characteristics, partition coefficient, large molecular size and fundamental physiology of the gastrointestinal tract (GIT). The gastrointestinal variables incorporate physiological properties of GIT fluids, gastric motility, gastric resistance time, presence of processing enzymes causing potential enzymatic degradation of the drug (*e.g.*, cytochrome P450) and interaction with efflux transporter systems like P-glycoprotein (P-gp), poor membrane permeability and intestinal efflux properties of GIT lumen [4].

Also, the irreversible expulsion of drugs by first-pass organs, including the digestive system, liver and lungs, are other impediments of drug retention. Likewise, despite their high permeability a large portion of the new chemical entities are commonly assimilated in the upper part of the small intestinal system, retention being significantly decreased after ileum. Therefore, if these drugs are not discharged in GIT, they will have less bioavailability. In this manner, the real difficulties of the pharmaceutical industries are the identification of the methodologies that reduce the oral retention of the drugs. Drug discharge is an essential and restricting parameter for the oral bioavailability of drugs, especially for drugs with less GIT solubility and high permeability. Enhancing the drug discharge profile of these drugs is conceivable to upgrade their bioavailability and diminish side effects [5, 6].

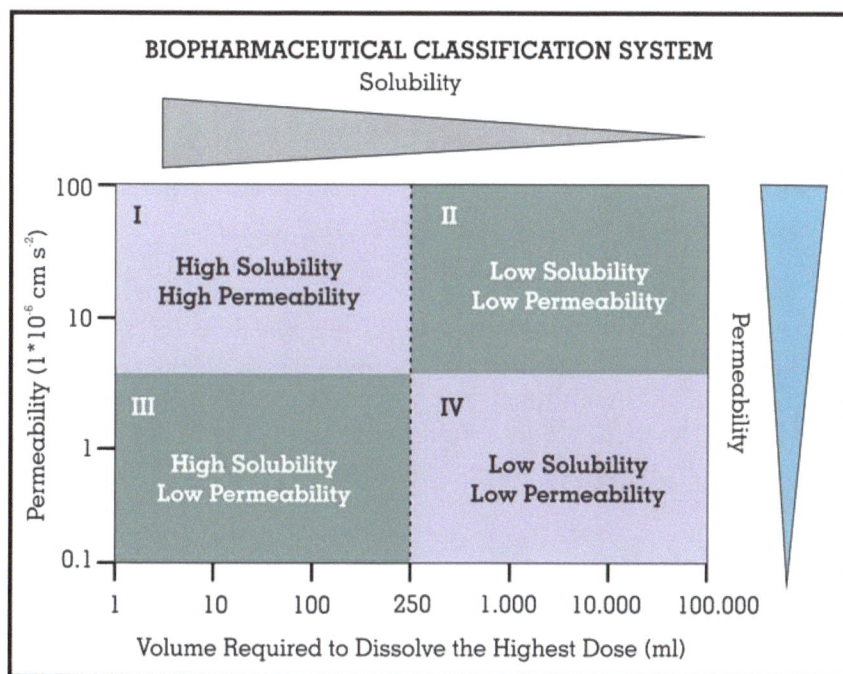

Fig. (1). Biopharmaceutical classification system.

Lipinski's rule of five has been broadly proposed as a qualitative prognostic model for assessment of the retention of ineffectively assimilated candidates. "The rule of 5" forecasts that poor retention or permeation occurs when more than 5H- bond donors are present, 10H-bond acceptors, molecular weight is higher than 500 and log P more than 5. Thus, *in vivo* estimation of new drug applicants in the creature is carried out to demonstrate the retention of drugs. Inadequately assimilated drugs represent a test to the formulation of researchers to create appropriate dosage form which can improve their bioavailability [7].

DRUG SOLUBILITY

Drug solubility is defined as the quantity of drug that passes it into solution when the equilibrium is achieved between the solute of drug in solution and any surplus, un-dissolved drug to create a saturated state solution at a predefined temperature.

The oral bioavailability relies upon different aspects like aqueous solubility, drug permeability, drug extent of dissolution, first-pass metabolism, pre-systemic metabolism and so forth. The majority of continuous reasons for less oral bioavailability are identified with less solubility and less permeability. The solubility and disintegration rate of the drugs are directly related with each other.

In this way, the bioavailability of a drug is subordinate to its dissolution and solubility parameters, as well as its membrane permeability and associated with degradation of the drug. There are various factors influencing solubilization such as the size of particle, temperature, pressure, molecular size, polarity, polymorphs and nature of solute & solvent.

REQUIREMENT FOR SOLUBILITY IMPROVEMENT

Drug retention through GIT can be restricted by a variety of variables. The major contributors among these are less water solubility and less permeability of the drug candidate through a membrane. When administered orally, it should first break down in gastric and additional intestinal fluids before it can penetrate the layers of GIT to arrive in blood circulation. Henceforth, two territories of pharmaceutical investigations need attention: one enhancing the bioavailability of orally administered drug candidates, and second is improving its solubility and extent of dissolution in water-soluble drugs. The BCS is a logical structure for arranging a drug compound based on its aqueous solubility and intestinal permeability [8].

APPROACHES TO ENHANCE ORAL BIOAVAILABILITY

The bioavailability of a drug is defined as the rate and extent to which a dissolved drug is assimilated and becomes available at its site of action. Various innovations can be utilized to improve solubility and among them, solid dispersion approach can be effectively helpful for the improvement of items from lab scale to commercial scale with a wide variety of powder qualities. Different pharmaceutical particle strategies are utilized to solve the issues related to the low water solubility of drug substances. The molecule approaches can be classified into two categories: traditional techniques and advanced particle strategies. Various approaches to enhance oral bioavailability are shown in Fig. (**2**).

The chemical modifications and formulation modifications are the few ways involved in enhancing the oral bioavailability. Chemical modification includes soluble pro-drug, salt formation and formulation modification comprises of physical changes like size reduction, crystal habit modification, complexation (*e.g.* with β-cyclodextrin), solubilization with co-solvents or surfactants, drug dispersion with carriers (*e.g.* eutectic mixture, solid dispersion and polymeric carriers like micro/nanoemulsions, self-emulsifying drug delivery systems (SEDDS), liposomes, solid lipid nanoparticles (SLNs) and nanostructured lipid carriers. The formulation approach is a superior option to a chemical modification approach, which may prompt the change in chemical structure and this may impact the pharmacological action. The achievement of the formulation modification approach is additionally restricted as they require the drugs to have particular properties, for instance, there should be an occurrence of β-cyclodextrin complexation, suitable molecular size and shape [9, 10].

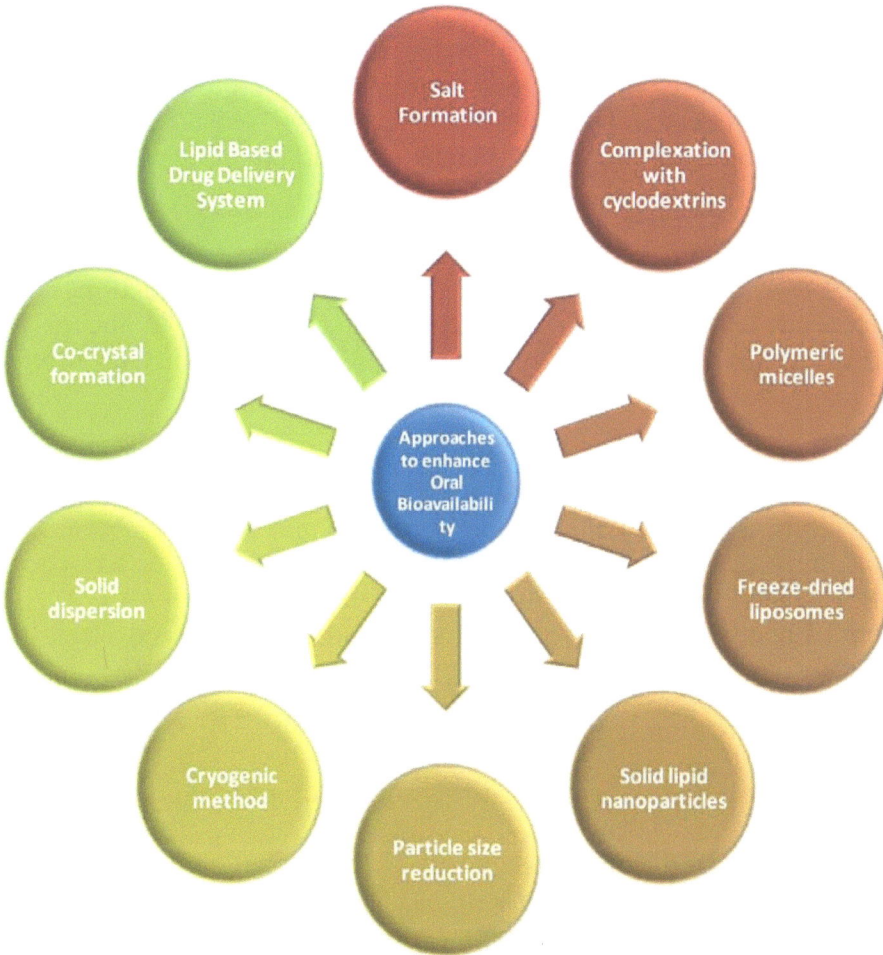

Fig. (2). Approaches to enhance oral bioavailability.

Current advanced particle technology can conquer the constraints of conventional strategies and more proficient techniques can be adopted for developing inadequately soluble drugs. The new techniques are created from traditional strategies where the fundamental guideline is the reduction of particle size for improving its solubility.

VARIOUS TECHNIQUES FOR IMPROVING BIOAVAILABILITY

Salt Formation

Salt formation is the most common approach for ionizable drugs to enhance solubility and dissolution of the drug. Salts are framed by proton exchange from acid to base. As indicated by the Henderson-Hassel Balch equation, the adjustment in pH profoundly impacts the aqueous solubility of an ionizable drug [8, 11].

Theoretically, the solubility of the weakly basic drug increases with diminishing pH at the pH range between its pKa and pH max. The expanded saturable solubility depends upon the dissolving area that participates in the greater disintegration rate by salt development. For example, the solubility of different diclofenac salts varies by a factor of 100 [10].

The dissolution rate of specific salt is generally unique with its parent candidate. Sodium and potassium salt of weak acids dissolve more hastily than an unadulterated salt. Limitation of the salt form is epigastric pain because of elevated alkalinity that leads to precipitation of atmospheric water and carbon dioxide, their reactivity, patient conformity and commercialization [12]. Salt development of neutral candidates isn't possible and weak acid and weak base salts may not always be practically possible to synthesize [13].

Cyclodextrins Based Complexes

Cyclodextrins are oligosaccharides consisting of a hydrophobic core cavity and hydrophilic external shell. There are various kinds of cyclodextrins based on the number of attached α-D-glucopyranose units. These are widely used in several pharmaceutical and nutraceutical compositions. They form an inclusion complex with poorly water-soluble drugs by entrapping them into their hydrophilic cavity as shown in Fig. (**3**). This leads to an increase in their solubility and results in improved bioavailability [14].

In pharmaceutical formulation methods, cyclodextrins are valuable solubilizers. The critical procedure related to the solubilization capability of cyclodextrins (CDs) is the incorporation of the developed complex, while the solubilization process may also be contributed by a non-inclusion complexation and supersaturation. There are a few strategies for the formation of a drug-cyclodextrin complex.

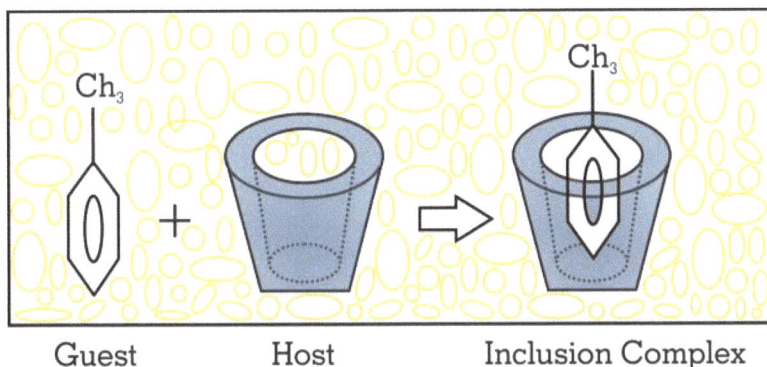

Fig. (3). Inclusion complexes of cyclodextrins.

Particle size, amount of complex development and the level of amorphous nature of the finished product result in the selection of planning technique which is vital when outlining drug cyclodextrin edifices. As far as toxicology and kinetics of solubility are concerned, CDs are well-thought-out in having advantage over organic solvents, drug entrapment efficacy and high drug loading capacity. After studying these investigations, it is concluded that CDs, particularly β-CD, can be an appropriate ingredient in pharmaceutical molecule innovation for enhancing the solubility of drugs with poor solubility [15, 16].

Jakab *et al.,* introduced baicalin and its CD complexes with enhanced bioavailability that have a bioactive phytopharmacon [17]. Complexation with cyclodextrin molecules isn't suitable for medicated molecules with no solubility in aqueous and organic solvents.

Gao *et al.,* formulated diuron loaded inclusion complex. They altered physicochemical properties by using *β*-CD that resulted in the enhancement of its herbicidal performance [18].

Saeid *et al.,* formulated melphalan loaded complex using β-CD macrocycle. They found that the 18:1 βCDg-Mel complex enhanced biological performance 2–3-times and lessen its concentration by approximately half for maximal inhibitory concentration [19].

Kontogiannidou *et al.,* formulated mucoadhesive tablets of piroxicam using co-evaporation method. They concluded that the drug discharge pattern was Me-CD > HP-β-CD > β-CD, whereas the *ex vivo* investigation demonstrated that chitosan-based tablets appreciably enhanced the transportation of drugs [20].

TECHNIQUES OF COMPLEXATION

Various techniques of complexation include:

Kneading Technique

The drug with the appropriate polymer in various proportions is placed in the mortar and triturated with a little amount of ethanol to prepare slurry. Gradually the drug is fused into slurry with consistent trituration. The slurry is then exposed to air drying at 250°C for 24hrs to obtain complex. The resulting complexes are pulverized, sift through 80 mesh and placed in a desiccator over fused $CaCl_2$.

Co-precipitation Technique

The drug is broken up in ethanol at moderate temperature and the reasonable carrier is disintegrated in filtered water. Distinctive molar proportions of drug and appropriate carriers are blended. The blend is mixed at a controlled temperature for 60 minutes and evaporation of the solvent is done. Pulverize resultant material, sift through 80 mesh and placed in desiccators.

Spray Drying

A spray dryer is utilized for the evaporation of drug and carrier solution in various proportions. The solutions are prepared by dissolving a drug in methanol and carrier in Milli Q water and the two solutions are then blended to obtain a clear solution. Then, the solution is introduced into the spray dryer for evaporation of the solvent and spray-dried blend of drug with carrier for 20-30 min, as shown in Fig. (**4**) [21, 22].

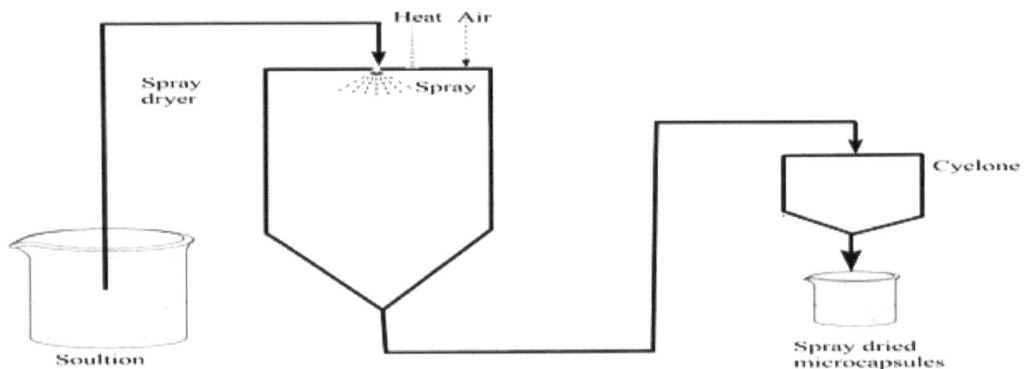

Fig. (4). Overview of spray drying process.

Zhang *et al.,* developed chitosan-based microspheres of *Panax notoginseng* extract, *Codonopsis* extract and *Atractylodes* extract with this technique. *In vitro* investigation showed a sustained release effect of the formulation. The particle diameter was 10.27 ± 1.05 μm with an encapsulation efficiency of $91.28 \pm 1.04\%$ [24].

Pohlen *et al.,* developed simvastatin loaded dry emulsion with this technique employing a mixture of caprylic, capric TG and 1-oleoyl-rac-glycerol, mannitol, HPMC, tween 20. This formulation resulted in suitable particle size distribution, good reconstitution ability and enhanced dissolution profile [25].

Wijiani *et al.,* developed curcumin-spray dried powder with self-assembled casein and sucrose, as a protectant. It showed a significant increase of drug solubility in presence of sucrose [26].

NOVEL FORMULATION APPROACHES FOR BIOAVAILABILITY ENHANCEMENT

There are some novel formulations for the bioavailability enhancement which are discussed below:

Polymeric Micelles

Polymeric micelles have risen as possible transporters for inadequately soluble drugs by making their inner core sluble and contributing appealing features such as a lesser size and an affinity to sidestep hunting by the mononuclear phagocyte system. In these systems, the lipophilic parts frame the center of the micelle, while the hydrophilic part forms the micelle's outer layer. The non-polar particles are solubilized inside the lipophilic part while polar compounds will be adsorbed on the surface of the micelles and molecules with moderate polarity will be dispersed with surfactants at an intermediate location as shown in Fig. (**5**) [27].

Drug loading is done by two different methods. The primary technique is the direct dissolution technique and the second technique is the solvent removal technique. The direct dissolution technique is a basic technique in which moderately hydrophobic block co-polymers are used along the drug in an aqueous solvent. Another technique is related to amphiphilic copolymers, which do not solubilize promptly in an aqueous phase and need an organic solvent for dissolving together. Micelle arrangement relies on the solvent removal process that can be performed by one of the few strategies like dialysis, solution casting, o/w emulsion and freeze-drying [28].

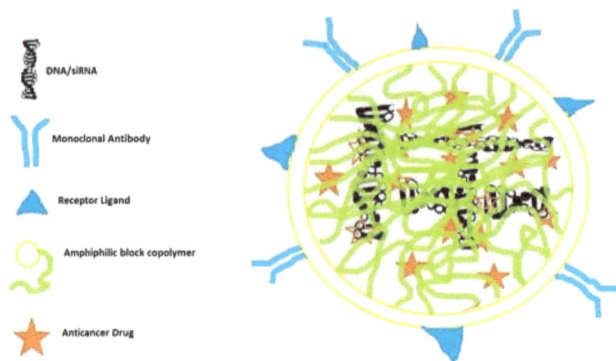

DNA/siRNA

Monoclonal Antibody

Receptor Ligand

Amphiphilic block copolymer

Anticancer Drug

Fig. (5). Polymeric micelles with entrapped anti-cancer drug**s**.

These are advanced systems that not only improve the aqueous solubility of the numerous lipophilic drugs, but are also applicable in drug targeting, preparing unstable drugs and lessening their adverse effects. Because of their extensive materialness to an enormous group of therapeutic candidates, drug-loading into polymeric micelles is a gifted particle technique for developing other inadequately soluble drugs in the future [29, 30].

Liposomes

These are vesicles of phospholipid (PL), involving a PL bilayer encompassing water partition and can break up lipophilic drugs in their lipid sphere. In the light of their biphasic attributes and assorted variety in formulation and administration, they propose a dynamic and versatile innovation for the improvement of drug solubility. Entrapment or encapsulation of drugs into liposomes changes pharmacokinetics and pharmacodynamics features of water-insoluble drugs and thus facilitates enormous improvement in the bioavailability and therapeutic value of drugs. During storage, poor stability is one of the genuine confinements with liposomes as drug delivery systems [31]. Thus, the freeze-drying method is utilized to obtain dry powders with upgraded stability while keeping the potency of added drugs in the liposomal formulations. This is a promising methodology for developing drugs with poor aqueous solubility and additionally upgrading the stability of liposomal formulations [32].

Abud *et al.*, evaluated a new formulation of sirolimus loaded liposome that resulted in negligible *in vitro* and *in vivo* toxicity in rabbit eyes [33].

Nkanga *et al.*, encapsulated an isoniazid-hydrazone-phthalocyanine conjugate (Pc-INH) complex system in γ-CD that was further transformed into liposomes using crude soybean lecithin by simple organic solvent-free and heating techniques [34].

Solid Lipid Nanoparticles (SLNs)

SLNs are colloidal drug transporter systems that resemble with nanoemulsions, however they consist of solid lipid such as glycerides or waxes (having a high melting point) as shown in Fig. (**6**).

Among different strategies for SLNs formulation, for example, High-pressure homogenization (HPH), solvent injection, solvent emulsification-evaporation, breaking of o/w microemulsion, double emulsion (w/o/w), high shear homogenization and ultrasound dispersion, HPH technique is thought to be the best strategy for SLN formulation. SLNs processed by HPH have many benefits of small particles, high dispersions content, removal of organic solvents and scale-up viability.

Their adhesive characteristics are responsible for increased bioavailability and reduced/minimize erratic assimilation. SLN innovation is invaluable over other systems because its probability of being formulated as drug discharge can be controlled. Their enhanced drug targeting on expanded drug stability, very low biotoxicity of the carrier and the possibility of consolidation of both hydrophilic and lipophilic drugs into the polymer are other advantages. In any case, certain impediments of SLN like less drug-loading capacities and stability issues amid storage or intake (gelation, increment in the particle size, drug removal from SLN) can't be dismissed [35].

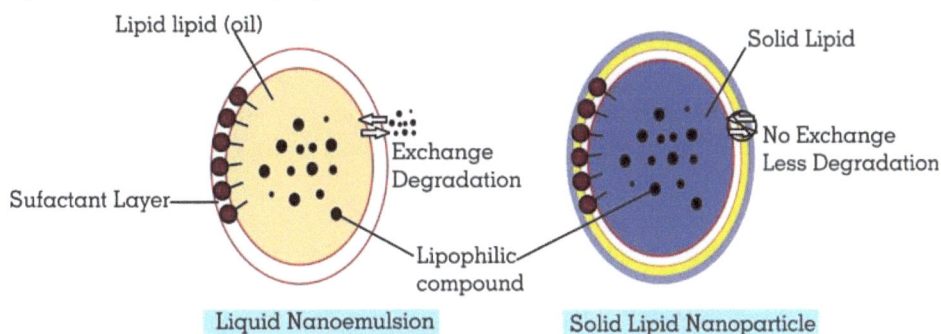

Fig. (**6**). Encapsulation of drugs in solid lipid nanoparticles.

Makoni *et al.,* formulated efavirenz-loaded SLN and nanostructured lipid carrier dispersions using HPH with glyceryl monostearate, transcutol HP and tween 80. The optimized formulations showed physical stability as aqueous dispersions [36].

Zielińska *et al.,* encapsulated bicyclic monoterpene of α-pinene into SLN by HPH. The optimized batch consists of α-pinene (1%), imwitor 900 K (4%) and poloxamer 188 (2.5%) that has a globule size of 136.7 nm with 0.170 of PDI and 0 mV of ZP [37].

Zhang *et al.,* formulated Resvasterol-SLN by emulsification-diffusion method. Resvasterol-SLN demonstrated the therapeutic potential for shielding of myocardium and lessened DOX-induced cardiotoxicity in mice [38].

Dendrimers

Dendrimers are large and highly branched polymers. These are synthesized, multi-branched polymeric compositions where the branches of the polymer originate from the core. Unique characteristics of dendrimers include their uniformly dispersed design, relatively spherical shape, adaptable surface composition, multi-valency, aqueous-solubility and available hydrophobic pockets/cavities at the interior which can encapsulate hydrophobes [39].

Gorzkiewicz *et al.,* developed dendriplexes using novel poly(lysine) dendrimers. They authenticated the hypothesis that the use of these polymers may permit a proficient method of siRNA transfer into the cells *in vitro* [40].

PARTICLE SIZE REDUCTION

The traditional strategies for this include mechanical micronization methods that are simple and helpful techniques to lessen drug particle size, result in incrementing in the surface area and hence improve solubility and dissolution of drugs. The traditional particle strategies are restricted for a few drugs because of their less efficiency, chemical alteration or degradation of drugs and bringing about non-uniform sized particles. The issue with micronization is chemical/thermal stability; numerous drugs may reduce bioactivity when micronization is done by conventional strategies [41]. As indicated by Williams *et al.,* particle size decrease to nano range includes two procedures to be specific 'bottom-up' and 'top-down strategy' [42].

Strategies

Two strategies reported in the literatures are discussed below:

1. Mechanical micronization
2. Engineered particle size control

Mechanical Micronization

A conventional method for particle size reduction is micronization and an ordinarily utilized technique for improving solubility of BCS class II drugs. The solubility and subsequent dissolution of the drug increments relatively by expanding surface region of drug particles. As indicated by the *Prandil Boundary Layer* equation, the reduction in thickness of the diffusion layer by reduction in particle size, especially less than 5μm, can bring about quickened dissolution [43].

Micronization does not expand the balance solubility of the drug itself; yet expanding the surface area, boosts the dissolution rate by drug proportion that results in dissolution or diffusion from a drug. Unadventurous, mechanical micronization like crushing, grinding and milling of formerly created bigger particles are used in pharmaceuticals for size reduction. Jet mill, ball mill and HPH are usually utilized for drugs. Jet mill (Energy mill) is the most favored micronization strategy for milling in a fluid [44]. These techniques have been used in different investigations to expand the dissolution and *in vivo* bioavailability by diminishing particle size and expanding the surface area of drugs. Micronization has been utilized effectively to upgrade the solubility of inadequately water-soluble drugs by utilizing jet milling, ball milling, HPH.

Jet Milling

For pharmaceutical powders, a fluid jet mill is used, which utilizes high-pressure air to achieve very fine granulating as shown in Fig. (**7**). It has a few points of interest in being a dry method; such as the particles of the micro-size range are obtained with uniform size of particles, lack of infectivity and appropriate for thermolabile drugs such as ibuprofen. salbutamol sulfate, fenoterol hydrobromide, amino acid, antibiotics, aspirin, guanylate, furosemide, penicillin, vitamin, deltamethrin, carbendazim, carbaryl, germicide, herbicide and fungicide [45].

Ball Milling

It is usually a cylindrical shape squashing gadget that is utilized for granulating powders of pharmaceutical-grade by revolving around a horizontal alliance. The gadget is incompletely loaded with substance to be crushed. In addition to the granulating medium, normally balls of stainless steel, ceramic, or flint pebbles are used as depicted in Fig. (**8**).

This instrument is utilized to formulate glass solutions by creating a single homogenous amorphous phase. The rate of dissolution was also established to be superior to spray-drying products of similar drugs. This proposes the appropriateness of this method to create homogenous amorphous formulations of inadequately soluble drugs. This can be vital to enhance the solubility of these types of drugs. Fenofibrate, indomethacin, cilostazol, ranitidine hydrochloride, a combination of griseofulvin and phenytoin, a combination of simvastatin and glipizide are micronized using a ball mill [43].

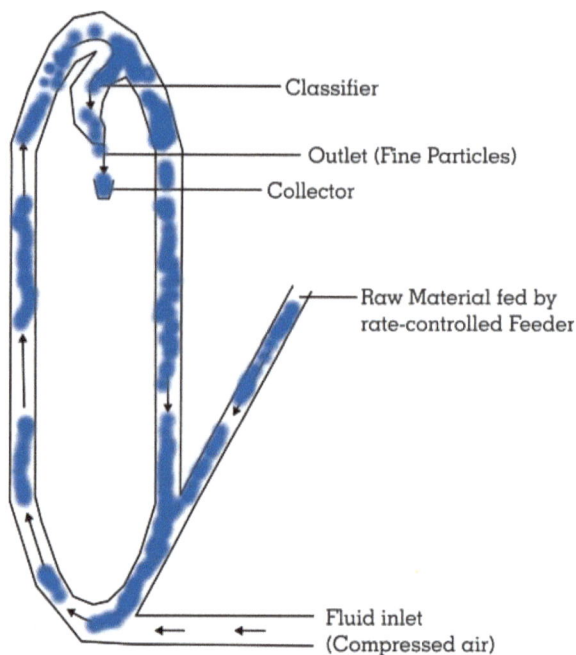

Fig. (7). Schematic diagram of a fluid energy mill.

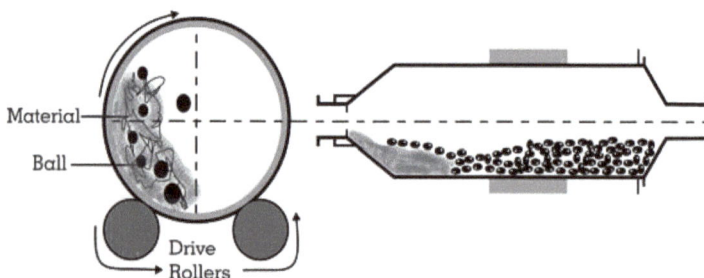

Fig. (8). Representation of a ball mill diagrammatically. The grinding media is prepared by the balls and drive rollers aid to rotate the milling chamber.

High-Pressure Homogenization

This is a top-down innovation, which is broadly utilized approach for developing nanosuspension of a drug that has PWS as shown in Fig. (**9**). Its utilization has been accounted for boostingthe extent of dissolution and bioavailability of several drugs by forceful size reduction to the nanoscale range. Likewise, it has been acknowledged to defeat the disadvantages of traditional size reducing techniques, for example, amorphization and polymorph change because of its high mechanical energy related to conventional milling methods. Due to this reason, it is especially beneficial for the comminution of drugs such as phenytoin and ketoprofen. In oral dose formulations, it has been generally utilized as a part of developing parental products of inadequately water-soluble drugs. This method is considered to be appropriate for parental products because of no danger of contamination and the high pressure can shield microbial contamination [46].

Guo *et al.,* formulated lotus seed starch, dispersed in deionized water with HPH and investigated the impact of HPH treatment on its physicochemical characteristics [47].

Makoni *et al.,* formulated efavirenz-loaded SLN and nanostructured lipid carrier dispersions using HPH with glyceryl monostearate, transcutol HP and tween 80. The optimized formulations showed physical stability as aqueous dispersions [36].

Zielińska *et al.,* encapsulated bicyclic monoterpene of α-pinene into SLN by HPH. The optimized batch consists of α-pinene (1%), imwitor 900 K (4%) and poloxamer 188 (2.5%) which has a globule size of 136.7 nm with 0.170 of PDI and 0 mV of ZP [37].

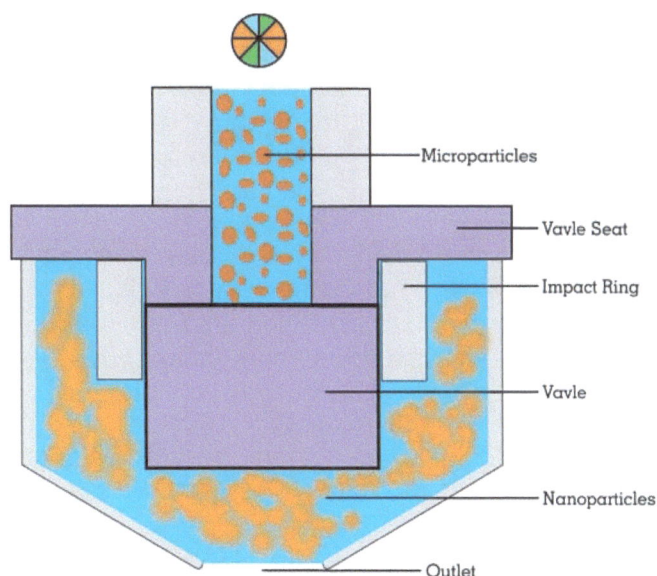

Fig. (9). Graphic representation of high-pressure homogenization method.

Engineered Particle Size Control

Conventional strategies for size reduction are generally known to have certain drawbacks *i.e.,* being less proficient because of high energy necessities, posturing dangers of heat, chemical degradation of drugs and the finished products have not uniform distribution of the particle size. Traditional milling strategies are thought to be unrestrained methods with restrictions to control size, shape, morphological features, surface characteristics and electrostatic charge and prompt non-uniform shapes of particle or even agglomerated particles as the final manufactured products. To beat these impediments and to explicitly control the features of particles, a few particle-building procedures have been created as an option and are used to deliver the required size of particles and precisely control their features. These advanced particle engineering techniques include cryogenic and crystal engineering processes that are advanced strategies for creating nanosized drug particles as an endeavor to diminish their particle size, upgrade solubility and dissolution [9].

Strategies of Cryogenic Method

Cryogenic Method

Cryogenic strategies are used to upgrade the rate of dissolution of drugs by making nanostructured amorphous particles of drugs with a high level of porosity at low-temperature. These innovations can be characterized by the type of injection gadget, area of nozzle and the components of cryogenic fluid. After the cryogenic process, drying is carried out using spray freeze drying, atmospheric freeze-drying, vacuum freeze-drying or lyophilization to obtain a dry powder. The atmospheric drying process is better than vacuum freeze-drying in the industry [8].

Craye *et al.,* explored the fabrication approach for co-amorphous simvastatin–lysine at 1:1 molar mixtures of sodium lauryl sulfate. This product can exhibit the enhanced physical stability of amorphous simvastatin [48].

Vadakkan *et al.,* used cryo-crystallization to convert isoniazid into inhalable particles. The crystals were dried using a lyophilization technique [49].

Spray Freezing onto Cryogenic Fluids

Briggs and Maxwell imagined this procedure of showering cryogenic liquids, solidifying onto solid to make them consolidated. In this technique, the drug and the polymer/carrier (maltose, MCC, HPMC) broken down in aqueous media and this solution atomized over the surface of a steaming agitated fluorocarbon refrigerant. Put probe of sonicator in the blended refrigerant to improve dispersion of solution.

Spray Freezing into Cryogenic Liquids

This particle engineering strategy is utilized to create amorphous nanostructured particles of the drug with a greater area of surface and high wettability. It adds direct liquid-liquid impingement among the automatized solution and cryogenic fluid to give exceptional microdroplets after atomization and therefore, a fundamentally quicker rate of freezing. Then, lyophilization of the cryogenic particles is carried out to acquire dry and micronized powders with excellent flow properties.

Spray Freezing into Vapor over Liquid

Freezing of drug solutions in cryogenic liquid vapors and ensuing expulsion of frozen solvent creates small drug particles with high wettability. Amid this process, the atomized beads frequently begin to freeze in the vapor phase before their contact with the cryogenic fluid. As the solvent freezes, the drug ends up being supersaturated in the unfrozen areas of the atomized bead, so fine drug particles are developed [46].

Ultra-rapid Freezing (URF)

This is a novel cryogenic innovation that makes nanostructured drug particles with the enormously improved surface region and required morphology of surface by utilizing solid cryogenic compounds. Utilization of drug solution for the solid surface of cryogenic substance prompts immediate freezing and ensuing lyophilization creates the micronized form of drug powder with enhanced solubility. URF impedes the separation of phase and the crystallization of the pharmaceutical fixings prompting familiarly blending, solid solutions and amorphous drug-carrier solid dispersions [50].

Crystal Engineering

It is another rising strategy for controlled crystallization that can be described as the development of a non-covalent bond between ionic or molecular constituents for the objective outline of solid-state configurations that may show fascinating electrical, magnetic and optical features. Metastable polymorphs, co-crystals, high energy amorphous and ultrafine particles are few advancements of it that enhance drug solubility through controlled crystallization procedures [51].

Co-crystals

It is another class of crystalline solids. When they are formulated into dosage form, they can give choices to improve features. Their development can be another option to form the salt in the case of neutral candidates or those who have feeble ionizable groups. The utilization of this technique expanded the dissolution extent up to 18 folds as compared with the homomeric crystalline type of a similar drug. Nanocrystals are crystalline, which are gaining prevalence in light of their capacity to build equilibrium solubility and dissolution rate. A few solvent-free drug crystal engineering strategies are recommended by indirect sonication, ultrasonic melt precipitation and wet milling [52].

Nicolov *et al.,* formulated betulinic acid loaded co-crystal using ascorbic acid as coformer in isopropyl alcohol to solve improve its low water solubility that results in its poor bioavailability [53].

Bagde *et al.,* formulated darunavir loaded co-crystals by cooling crystallization method using succinic acid as coformer [54].

Sopyan *et al.,* developed simvastatin loaded co-crystals by co-crystallization using nicotinamide as coformer by solvent evaporation to improve its solubility [55].

Nanoparticles

Nanotechnology is a new field of science that takes the benefits of peculiar features of matter at the nanoscale. Nano-sizing is defined as diminishing the particle size of the active pharmaceutical ingredients (API) to the sub-micron range of 100-200 nm. This prompts a huge increment in the rate of dissolution of the API, which like this prompts a generous increment in the bioavailability [31]. The solid API dissolution rate is related to the surface area accessible for dissolution as depicted by the Noyes-Whitney equation:

$$dx/dt = A.D (Cs-Cb)/(V.h)$$

Where dx/dt = rate of dissolution,

D= diffusion coefficient,

A= surface area of dissolving particle,

$Cs-Cb$ = conc. gradient for the diffusion of drug,

V= volume of dissolution medium,

h = effective boundary layer thickness.

Their vehicles appreciably decline side-effects of drugs (mainly anti-cancer) by enhancing their aqueous solubility and diminishing the overall required dose. Hybrid nanoparticles, gold nanoparticles, folate-targeting nanoparticles, chitosan based hybrid nanoparticles and lipid-polymer hybrid nanoparticles are novel advancements in nanoparticles.

Solid Dispersion (SD)

It is a precious pharmaceutical method for improving the rate of dissolution, retention and therapeutic potential of API in the dosage form. This comprises of a solid item with a hydrophilic polymer lattice and a hydrophobic drug. The most usually utilized hydrophilic polymers for SDs are povidone, PEGs and so on and surfactants like polysorbate-80, docusate sodium, Myrj-52 and so on. Utilizing reasonable hydrophilic polymers such as povidone with celecoxib and gelucire for ritonavir resulted in enhancement of their solubility by using this technique [8, 56].

TECHNIQUES OF SOLID DISPERSION

Various techniques of SD are discussed below:

Fusion (melt) Technique

This technique precisely measures quantities of the carrier (s) placed in a container of aluminum on a hot plate and liquefied with consistent mixing at 60°C. A precisely measured quantity of active drug is added into it with continuous blending to assure homogeneity. The blend is warmed until a clear uniform melt is acquired. Then, the container is removed from the hot plate and is permitted to cool [57 - 59].

Solvent Technique

In this technique, precisely measured quantities of active drug and carrier(s) are dissolved in the least amounts of solvent in a round-bottom flask. A rotary evaporator is utilized to remove/evaporate the solvent. Thus, the product is shifted on the container and permitted to dry at normal temperature [60].

Dropping Technique

Pipette out drug-carrier mixture and after that fall down onto a plate, where it solidifies into round particles. The shape and size of the particles can be influenced by various parameters such as the consistency of melting and pipette size. Since thickness is exceptionally temperature subordinate, it is vital to modify the temperature to ensure that a spherical shape is obtained when the melted mixture falls onto the plate [58].

Co-crystal Formation

Pharmaceutical co-crystal is made out of an API and inert excipients (co-crystal former) in a stoichiometric proportion. The API and co-crystal former require hydrogen bonding to frame a stable co-crystal. For the most part, ΔpKa is one of the reliable pointers for recognizing salts and co-crystal. AMG-517 is a free base that is crystallized with sorbic acid that demonstrated a higher rate of dissolution in a simulated fasted state and 9.4-folds improvement in AUC was found [6].

Supercritical Fluid Recrystallization (SCF)

These fluids contain features of both gases and liquids. Carbon dioxide is the best example of this. These are exceptionally compressible at critical temperatures and permits modification in density and mass transport qualities thatdecides its solvent power because of the direct alteration in pressure. As the drugs is solubilized inside SCF, they can be recrystallized with diminished molecule size of drug [61 - 63].

Sonocrystallisation

In this technique, liquid solvents and anti-solvents are additionally utilized to lessen particle size effectively. This is an advanced strategy for particle size diminishment based on crystallization by utilizing ultrasound of frequency 20–100 kHz for initiating this process. It improves nucleation rate as well as compelling methods for size reduction and control uniformity in the particle size distribution. In the majority of applications, 20 kHz-5 MHz range of frequency is used [50, 64].

Liquisolid Technique

The liquisolid method is an advanced idea in which fluid might be altered into a free-flowing, promptly compressible and dry powder by straightforward physical mixing with chosen polymer and coating substance. The fluid part which can be a liquid drug, suspension or solution is mixed in an appropriate non-volatile liquid vehicle which is added into a porous carrier substance. Once the carrier is saturated with liquid, a liquid layer is framed on the molecule surface which is right away adsorbed by coating particles that are fine. Accordingly, a dry, free streaming and compressible powder is obtained [65 - 70].

Formation of Inclusion Complex

Among solubility upgrade strategies, this strategy has been utilized to improve solubility, the extent of dissolution and bioavailability of drugs. These are prepared by the inclusion of the non-polar compounds or non-polar area of one molecule (known as the visitor) into the hole of other compounds or cavity of a molecule (called as host) [71 - 73]. CDs are the most commonly utilized as host molecules. The cavity of the host must be sufficiently extensive to oblige visitors and sufficiently little to eradicate water, with the goal that the aggregate makes a contact between the water and the non-polar region to reduce the non-polar region of the host and the visitor [74]. Solid inclusion complexes are formulated by various techniques which are discussed below:

Kneading Method

This technique depends upon the saturation of CDs with a small quantity of water or hydroalcoholic solution for change over into a paste. Then, the drug is incorporated into paste and kneading is done for a predefined time. Then, the kneaded blend is dried and sifted through a mesh if essential. In the research lab, this can be accomplished by utilizing a pestle, mortar and extruders. It is a widely recognized and straightforward strategy utilized to formulate inclusion complexes; furthermore, it introduces minimal effort of production [75 - 77].

Lyophilization/Freeze-Drying Technique

Keeping in mind the end goal to obtain a porous and amorphous powder with a high degree of interface among drug and CD, this method is considered as reasonable. In this method, the solvent system from the solution is wiped out through an essential freezing and consequent drying of the solution containing both drug and CD at decreased pressure. This technique can be effectively utilized for thermolabile substances to produce complex forms. The confinements of this strategy are utilizing a particular apparatus, consuming more time and giving the poor flow of powdered products. This technique is the best alternative for solvent evaporation and molecular blending of drugs with carriers in a common solvent. Typhoid vaccine, live measles virus vaccine, meningococcal polysaccharide vaccine groups A and C combined and interferon-α are the products that are prepared by this technique [50, 78].

Microwave Irradiation Method

This system includes microwave illumination reactions among drug and chelating agents utilizing an oven. The drug and CDs in fixed molar proportions are solubilized in a mixture of organic solvent and water to a predetermined extent into an RBF. The blend is reacted in the microwave oven for a brief time of around 1-2 minutes at 60°C. After completion of the reaction, a sufficient quantity of the solvent mixture is incorporated into the reaction blend to evacuate the remaining, uncomplexed free drug and CD. The powder is isolated utilizing filter paper and dried in a vacuum oven [50].

Self-micro Emulsifying Drug Delivery Systems (SMEDDS)

SMEDDS utilizes the idea of *in situ* development of emulsion in the GI tract. SEDDS and SMEDDS are the isotropic mixtures of oil and surfactant that create o/w microemulsions on gentle agitation within the existence of water. The inadequately soluble drug can be dissolved in the blend which is broadly called preconcentrate. These advanced colloidal preparations on oral ingestion behave o/w microemulsion. In contrast with microemulsions, they appeared to enhance the physical stability of the formulation [79].

Kim *et al.,* exploited methotrexate-loaded solid-SMEDDS with enhanced bioavailability and photostability [80].

Desai *et al.,* encapsulated a unique low-dose combination in SMEDDS form (loratadine with sulforaphane) that demonstrated appreciably improved chemopreventive potential [81].

Verma *et al.,* developed microemulsion preconcentrates of telmisartan to improve its solubility that helps in enhancement of oral bioavailability profile using D-optimal mixture design [82].

Verma *et al.,* developed preconcentrates of nano-emulsions for the candesartan cilexetil to improve its pharmacodynamic impact and to avoid the food effect [83].

Particle technologies, the method used and example drugs used are shown in Table **1** [35, 62, 63].

Table 1. Particle technologies, the method and examples of drugs used.

Name of Technology	Method	Drugs Used
Mechanical micronization	Jet mill	Cilostazol, ibuprofen
	Ball mill	Danazol, dypyridamole, carbamazepine
	High-pressure homogenization	Carbamazepine, prednisolone
Novel particle engineering	Cryogenic spraying process/spray	Danazol
	Freezing into liquid	Carbamazepine
	Crystal engineering	Itrazonazole, glibenclamide

(Table 1) cont.....

Name of Technology	Method	Drugs Used
Solidification of SEDDS	Spray drying, *in situ* salt formation, solidification using polymers	Nimodipin, meloxicam, crucumin, ibuprofen, Dexibuprofen, docetaxel, flurbiprofen, fenofibrate
Complex formation	Kneading, co-precipitation	Praziquantel, clotrimazole, celecoxib
Polymeric micelles	Freeze-drying, dialysis	Celecoxib, amphotericin B, cyclosporine, quercetin
Freeze-dried liposomes	Freeze-drying	Paclitaxel, Sirolomus
SLNs	HPH, solvent emulsification-evaporation/diffusion	Levofloxacin-doxycycline, cilnidipine
Spray drying	-	Ascorbic acid, simvastatin

The choice of reasonable technique for solubility upgrade has relied upon drug features like melting point, solubility, chemical nature, physical nature, pharmacokinetic aspects and so on.

The different systems enrolled in this section are utilized as a combination for solubility upgradation of inadequately water-soluble drugs; however, the solubility change mostly relies upon selecting a justifiable technique.

CONSENT FOR PUBLICATION

Not applicable.

CONFLICT OF INTEREST

The author declares no conflict of interest, financial or otherwise.

ACKNOWLEDGEMENTS

Declared none.

REFERENCES

[1]   Padia N, Shukla A, Shelat P. Development and characterization of fenofibrate self-microemulsifying drug delivery system (SMEDDS) for bioavailability enhancement. Bull Pharm Res 2015; 5(2): 59-69.

[2]   Alexander A. A review on novel therapeutic strategies for the enhancement of solubility for hydrophobic drugs through lipid and surfactant-based self-microemulsifying drug delivery system: a novel approach. Am J Drug Disc Dev 2012; 2(4): 143-83.
      [http://dx.doi.org/10.3923/ajdd.2012.143.183]

[3]   Aınaoui A, Vergnaud JM. Modeling the plasma drug level with oral controlled release dosage forms with lipidic Gelucire. Int J Pharm 1998; 169(2): 155-62.

[http://dx.doi.org/10.1016/S0378-5173(98)00105-7]

[4]   Loh ZH, Samanta AK, Heng PW. Overview of milling techniques for improving the solubility of poorly water-soluble drugs. Asian J Pharm Sci 2015; 10(4): 255-74.
[http://dx.doi.org/10.1016/j.ajps.2014.12.006]

[5]   Badawy SI, Gray DB, Zhao F, Sun D, Schuster AE, Hussain MA. Formulation of solid dosage forms to overcome gastric pH interaction of the factor Xa inhibitor, BMS-561389. Pharm Res 2006; 23(5): 989-96.
[http://dx.doi.org/10.1007/s11095-006-9899-z] [PMID: 16715389]

[6]   Bak A, Gore A, Yanez E, *et al.* The co-crystal approach to improve the exposure of a water-insoluble compound: AMG 517 sorbic acid co-crystal characterization and pharmacokinetics. J Pharm Sci 2008; 97(9): 3942-56.
[http://dx.doi.org/10.1002/jps.21280] [PMID: 18214948]

[7]   Lipinski CA, Lombardo F, Dominy BW, Feeney PJ. Experimental and computational approaches to estimate solubility and permeability in drug discovery and development settings. Adv Drug Deliv Rev 2001; 46(1-3): 3-26.
[http://dx.doi.org/10.1016/S0169-409X(00)00129-0] [PMID: 11259830]

[8]   Savjani KT, Gajjar AK, Savjani JK. Drug solubility: importance and enhancement techniques. ISRN Pharm 2012; 2012(1)195727
[PMID: 22830056]

[9]   Khadka P, Ro J, Kim H, *et al.* Pharmaceutical particle technologies: An approach to improve drug solubility, dissolution and bioavailability. Asian J Pharm Sci 2014; 9(6): 304-16.
[http://dx.doi.org/10.1016/j.ajps.2014.05.005]

[10]   Serajuddin AT. Salt formation to improve drug solubility. Adv Drug Deliv Rev 2007; 59(7): 603-16.
[http://dx.doi.org/10.1016/j.addr.2007.05.010] [PMID: 17619064]

[11]   Avdeef A. Solubility of sparingly-soluble ionizable drugs. Adv Drug Deliv Rev 2007; 59(7): 568-90.
[http://dx.doi.org/10.1016/j.addr.2007.05.008] [PMID: 17644216]

[12]   Jatwani S, Rana AC, Singh G, Aggarwal G. An overview on solubility enhancement techniques for poorly soluble drugs and solid dispersion as an eminent strategic approach. Int J Pharm Sci Res 2012; 3: 942-56.

[13]   Dwichandra Putra O, Umeda D, Fujita E, *et al.* Solubility improvement of benexate through salt formation using artificial sweetener. Pharmaceutics 2018; 10(2): 1-12.
[http://dx.doi.org/10.3390/pharmaceutics10020064] [PMID: 29861459]

[14]   Brewster ME, Loftsson T. Cyclodextrins as pharmaceutical solubilizers. Adv Drug Deliv Rev 2007; 59(7): 645-66.
[http://dx.doi.org/10.1016/j.addr.2007.05.012] [PMID: 17601630]

[15]   Singh A, Worku ZA, Van den Mooter G. Oral formulation strategies to improve solubility of poorly water-soluble drugs. Expert Opin Drug Deliv 2011; 8(10): 1361-78.
[http://dx.doi.org/10.1517/17425247.2011.606808] [PMID: 21810062]

[16]   Carrier RL, Miller LA, Ahmed I. The utility of cyclodextrins for enhancing oral bioavailability. J Control Release 2007; 123(2): 78-99.
[http://dx.doi.org/10.1016/j.jconrel.2007.07.018] [PMID: 17888540]

[17]   Jakab G, Bogdán D, Mazák K, *et al.* Physicochemical profiling of baicalin along with the development and characterization of cyclodextrin inclusion complexes. AAPS PharmSciTech 2019; 20(8): 314-37.
[http://dx.doi.org/10.1208/s12249-019-1525-6] [PMID: 31529175]

[18]   Gao S, Jiang JY, Liu YY, *et al.* Enhanced solubility, stability and herbicidal activity of the herbicide diuron by complex formation with β-cyclodextrin. Polymers (Basel) 2019; 11(9): 1396-8.
[http://dx.doi.org/10.3390/polym11091396] [PMID: 31450656]

[19]   Mohammed-Saeid W, Karoyo AH, Verrall RE, Wilson LD, Badea I. Inclusion complexes of melphalan with gemini-conjugated β- cyclodextrin: Physicochemical properties and chemotherapeutic efficacy in *in-vitro* tumor models. Pharmaceutics 2019; 11(9): 427-49.
      [http://dx.doi.org/10.3390/pharmaceutics11090427] [PMID: 31443452]

[20]   Kontogiannidou E, Ferrari M, Deligianni AD, *et al. In vitro* and *ex vivo* evaluation of tablets containing piroxicam-cyclodextrin complexes for buccal delivery. Pharmaceutics 2019; 11(8): 398-15.
      [http://dx.doi.org/10.3390/pharmaceutics11080398] [PMID: 31398833]

[21]   Pawar A. Novel techniques for solubility, dissolution rate and bioavailability enhancement of class II and IV drugs. Asian J Biomed Pharma Sci 2012; 2(13): 9-20.

[22]   Kaushik D, Dureja H. Spray-dried microspheres of roxithromycin for formulating into dispersible tablets using central composite design. Appl Clin Res Clin Trials Regul Aff 2016; 3(2): 127-37.
      [http://dx.doi.org/10.2174/2213476X03666160727123840]

[23]   Kaushik D, Dureja H. Taste masking of bitter pharmaceuticals by spray drying technique. J Chem Pharm Res 2015; 7(4): 950-6.

[24]   Zhang ZL, Li LJ, Sun D, *et al.* Preparation and properties of chitosan-based microspheres by spray drying. Food Sci Nutr 2020; 8(4): 1933-41.
      [http://dx.doi.org/10.1002/fsn3.1479] [PMID: 32328259]

[25]   Pohlen M, Lavrič Z, Prestidge C, Dreu R. Preparation, physicochemical characterisation and doe optimisation of a spray-dried dry emulsion platform for delivery of a poorly soluble drug, simvastatin. AAPS PharmSciTech 2020; 21(4): 119.
      [http://dx.doi.org/10.1208/s12249-020-01651-x] [PMID: 32318974]

[26]   Wijiani N, Isadiartuti D, Rijal MAS, Yusuf H. characterization and dissolution study of micellar curcumin-spray dried powder for oral delivery. Int J Nanomedicine 2020; 15: 1787-96.
      [http://dx.doi.org/10.2147/IJN.S245050] [PMID: 32214811]

[27]   Gaucher G, Dufresne MH, Sant VP, Kang N, Maysinger D, Leroux JC. Block copolymer micelles: preparation, characterization and application in drug delivery. J Control Release 2005; 109(1-3): 169-88.
      [http://dx.doi.org/10.1016/j.jconrel.2005.09.034] [PMID: 16289422]

[28]   Kwon GS, Okano T. Polymeric micelles as new drug carriers. Adv Drug Deliv Rev 1996; 21(2): 107-16.
      [http://dx.doi.org/10.1016/S0169-409X(96)00401-2]

[29]   Yu BG, Okano T, Kataoka K, Kwon G. 1998.

[30]   Dangi JS, Vyas SP, Dixit VK. The role of mixed micelles in drug delivery. I. Solubilization. Drug Dev Ind Pharm 1998; 24(7): 681-4.
      [http://dx.doi.org/10.3109/03639049809082372] [PMID: 9876515]

[31]   Yang T, Cui FD, Choi MK, *et al.* Liposome formulation of paclitaxel with enhanced solubility and stability. Drug Deliv 2007; 14(5): 301-8.
      [http://dx.doi.org/10.1080/10717540601098799] [PMID: 17613018]

[32]   Ghanbarzadeh S, Valizadeh H, Zakeri-Milani P. The effects of lyophilization on the physico-chemical stability of sirolimus liposomes. Adv Pharm Bull 2013; 3(1): 25-9.
      [PMID: 24312808]

[33]   Abud MB, Louzada RN, Isaac DLC, *et al.* Encapsulation of isoniazid-conjugated phthalocyanine-i--cyclodextrin-in-liposomes using heating method. Int J Retina Vitreous 2019; 5: 35-54.
      [http://dx.doi.org/10.1186/s40942-019-0186-7] [PMID: 31572617]

[34]   Nkanga CI, Krause RWM. Short term stability testing of efavirenz-loaded solid lipid nanoparticle (SLN) and nanostructured lipid carrier (NLC) dispersions. Sci Rep 2019; 9: 11485-2.
      [http://dx.doi.org/10.1038/s41598-019-47991-y] [PMID: 31391517]

[35]   Müller RH, Mäder K, Gohla S. Solid lipid nanoparticles (SLN) for controlled drug delivery - a review of the state of the art. Eur J Pharm Biopharm 2000; 50(1): 161-77.
[http://dx.doi.org/10.1016/S0939-6411(00)00087-4] [PMID: 10840199]

[36]   Makoni PA, Kasongo KW, Walker RB. Development and optimization of alpha-pinene-loaded solid lipid nanoparticles (SLN) using experimental factorial design and dispersion analysis. Pharmaceutics 2019; 11(8): 397-24.
[http://dx.doi.org/10.3390/pharmaceutics11080397] [PMID: 31398820]

[37]   Zielińska A, Ferreira NR, Durazzo A, *et al.* Resveratrol solid lipid nanoparticles to trigger credible inhibition of doxorubicin cardiotoxicity. Molecules 2019; 24(15): 2683-107.
[PMID: 31344802]

[38]   Zhang L, Zhu K, Zeng H, *et al.* Physicochemical properties and digestion of lotus seed starch under high-pressure homogenization. Int J Nanomedicine 2019; 14: 6061-71.
[http://dx.doi.org/10.2147/IJN.S211130] [PMID: 31534336]

[39]   Choudhary S, Gupta L, Rani S, Dave K, Gupta U. Sarita Rani, Gupta U. Impact of dendrimers on solubility of hydrophobic drug molecules. Front Pharmacol 2017; 8: 261.
[http://dx.doi.org/10.3389/fphar.2017.00261] [PMID: 28559844]

[40]   Gorzkiewicz M, Kopeć O, Janaszewska A, *et al.* Poly(lysine) dendrimers form complexes with SiRNA and provide its efficient uptake by myeloid cells: Model studies for therapeutic nucleic acid delivery. Int J Mol Sci 2020; 21(9)E3138
[http://dx.doi.org/10.3390/ijms21093138] [PMID: 32365579]

[41]   Salazar J, Müller RH, Möschwitzer JP. Combinative particle size reduction technologies for the production of drug nanocrystals. J Pharm (Cairo) 2014; 2014(4)265754
[http://dx.doi.org/10.1155/2014/265754] [PMID: 26556191]

[42]   Williams HD, Trevaskis NL, Charman SA, *et al.* Strategies to address low drug solubility in discovery and development. Pharmacol Rev 2013; 65(1): 315-499.
[http://dx.doi.org/10.1124/pr.112.005660] [PMID: 23383426]

[43]   Junyaprasert VB, Morakul B. Nanocrystals for enhancement of oral bioavailability of poorly water-soluble drugs. Asian J Pharm Sci 2015; 10(1): 13-23.
[http://dx.doi.org/10.1016/j.ajps.2014.08.005]

[44]   Rasenack N, Müller BW. Micron-size drug particles: common and novel micronization techniques. Pharm Dev Technol 2004; 9(1): 1-13.
[http://dx.doi.org/10.1081/PDT-120027417] [PMID: 15000462]

[45]   Midoux N, Hošek P, Pailleres L, Authelin JR. Micronization of pharmaceutical substances in a spiral jet mill. Powder Technol 1999; 104(2): 113-20.
[http://dx.doi.org/10.1016/S0032-5910(99)00052-2]

[46]   Rahman MM, Khalipha ABR, Ahmed A, Rafshanjani MA, Haque S.

[47]   Guo Z, Zhao B, Chen L, Zheng B. Cocrystal formation of betulinic acid and ascorbic acid: synthesis, physico-chemical assessment, antioxidant and antiproliferative activity. Nutrients 2019; 11(2): 371-99.
[http://dx.doi.org/10.3390/nu11020371] [PMID: 30754686]

[48]   Craye G, Löbmann K, Grohganz H, Rades T, Laitinen R. Characterization of amorphous and co-amorphous simvastatin formulations prepared by spray drying. Molecules 2015; 20(12): 21532-48.
[http://dx.doi.org/10.3390/molecules201219784] [PMID: 26633346]

[49]   Vadakkan MV, Kumar GSV. Cryo-crystallization under a partial anti-solvent environment as a facile technology for dry powder inhalation development. Int J Nanomedicine 2019; 14: 6061-71.

[50]   Patil MS, Godse SZ, Saudagar RB. Solubility enhancement by various techniques: an overview. World J Pharm Pharm Sci 2016; 2(6): 4558-72.

[51]   Deerle D, Patel J, Yeole D, *et al.* Particle engineering techniques to enhance dissolution of poorly

water-soluble drugs. Int J Curr Pharm Res 2010; 2: 10-5.

[52]   Blagden N, de Matas M, Gavan PT, York P. Crystal engineering of active pharmaceutical ingredients to improve solubility and dissolution rates. Adv Drug Deliv Rev 2007; 59(7): 617-30.
[http://dx.doi.org/10.1016/j.addr.2007.05.011] [PMID: 17597252]

[53]   Nicolov M, Ghiulai RM, Voicu M, Mioc M, Duse AO. Frontiers (Boulder) 2019; 4(12): 44-56.

[54]   Bagde SA, Upadhye KP, Dixit GR, Bakhle SS. Formulation and evaluation of co-crystals of poorly water-soluble drug. Int J Pharm Sci Res 2019; 4(22): 22-44.

[55]   Sopyan I, Fudholi A, Muchtaridi M, Sari SP. Simvastatin-nicotinamide co-crystal: Design, preparation and preliminary characterization. Trop J Pharm Res 2017; 16(2): 297-03.
[http://dx.doi.org/10.4314/tjpr.v16i2.6]

[56]   Kumar S, Singh P. Various techniques for solubility enhancement: An overview. Pharma Innov 2016; 5 (1 Part A): 23-38.

[57]   Habib MJ. Pharmaceutical solid dispersion technology. Lancaster, Pennsylvania, U.S.A.: Technomic Publishing Company, Inc. 2001; pp. 1-36.

[58]   Vasconcelos T, Sarmento B, Costa P. Solid dispersions as strategy to improve oral bioavailability of poor water soluble drugs. Drug Discov Today 2007; 12(23-24): 1068-75.
[http://dx.doi.org/10.1016/j.drudis.2007.09.005] [PMID: 18061887]

[59]   Vemula VR, Lagishetty V, Lingala S. Solubility enhancement techniques. Int J Pharm Sci Rev Res 2010; 5(1): 41-51.

[60]   Mogal SA, Gurjar PN, Yamgar DS, Kamod AC. Solid dispersion technique for improving solubility of some poorly soluble drugs. Der Pharm Lettr 2012; 4: 1574-86.

[61]   Nikghal LA, Singh G, Singh G, Kahkeshan KF. Solid dispersion: Methods and polymers to increase the solubility of poorly soluble drugs. J Appl Pharm Sci 2012; 2: 170-85.

[62]   Mohanachandran PS, Sindhumol PG, Kiran TS. Enhancement of solubility and dissolution rate: An overview. Int J of Compehensive Pharm 2010; 1(4): 1-10.

[63]   Khalid ME, Ahmed M. Samy, Mohamed I. Formulation and evaluation of Rofecoxib liquisolid tablets. Int J Pharm Sci Rev Res 2010; 3(1): 135-42.

[64]   Chandel P, Raj K, Kapoor A. Liquisolid technique: an approach for enhancement of solubility. J Drug Deliv Ther 2013; 3(4): 131-7.
[http://dx.doi.org/10.22270/jddt.v3i4.556]

[65]   Gavali SM, Pacharane SS, Sankpal SV, Jadhav KR, Kadam VJ. Liquisolid Compact: A new technique for enhancement of drug dissolution. Int J Res Pharm Chem 2011; 1(3): 705-13.

[66]   Syed IM, Pavani E. The Liquisolid technique based drug delivery system. Int J Pharm Sci Drug Res 2012; 4(2): 88-96.

[67]   Vajir S. Liquisolid Compact: A novel approach to enhance bioavailability of poorly soluble drug. Int J Pharm 2012; 2(3): 586-90.

[68]   Spiridon Spireas, Bolton SM, Bolton SM. Liquisolids: Liquisolid system and methods of preparing the same. United States Patent 1998.

[69]   Godse SZ, Patil MS, Kothavade SM, Saudagar RB. Techniques for solubility enhancement of hydrophobic drugs: A review J Adv Pharm Edu & Res 2013.

[70]   Rawat S, Derle DV, Parve BS, Shinde PR. Self-emulsifying drug delivery system (SEDDS): A method for bioavailability enhancement. Int J Pharm Chem Biol Sci 2014; 4: 479-94.

[71]   Sharma PH, Kalasare SN, Damania H. Poorly soluble drugs - A challenge in drug delivery system. Eur J Pharm Med Res 2015; 2: 484-02.

[72]   Akhilesh D, Mehta H, Prabhakara P, Kamath JV. Enhancement of solubility by complexation with

cyclodextrin and nanocrystallisation. Int Res J Pharma 2012; 3(5): 100-5.

[73]   Kumar PD, Arora V. Solid dispersion: A review. J Pharm Scientific Innov 2012; 1(3): 28-35.

[74]   Reddy N, Reddy A, Srinivasan S. Review on: Better solubility enhancement of poorly water-soluble drugs. Int J Invent Pharm Sci 2013; 1(4): 267-73.

[75]   Kim EJ, Chun MK, Jang JS, Lee IH, Lee KR, Choi HK. Preparation of a solid dispersion of felodipine using a solvent wetting method. Eur J Pharm Biopharm 2006; 64(2): 200-5.
[http://dx.doi.org/10.1016/j.ejpb.2006.04.001] [PMID: 16750355]

[76]   Devil NKD, Rani AP, Javed M, Kumar KS, Kaushik J. Sowjanya. Cyclodextrins in pharmacy-An overview. Pharmacophore 2010; 1(3): 155-65.

[77]   Sareen S, Mathew G, Joseph L. Improvement in solubility of poor water-soluble drugs by solid dispersion. Int J Pharm Investig 2012; 2(1): 12-7.
[http://dx.doi.org/10.4103/2230-973X.96921] [PMID: 23071955]

[78]   Kumar SK, Sushma M, Raju PY. Dissolution enhancement of poorly soluble drugs by using complexation technique: A review. J Pharm Sci Res 2013; 5: 120-34.

[79]   Verma R, Mittal V, Kaushik D. Self-microemulsifying drug delivery system: A vital approach for bioavailability enhancement. Int J Chemtech Res 2017; 10(7): 515-28.

[80]   Kim DS, Cho JH, Park JH, *et al.* Self-microemulsifying drug delivery system (SMEDDS) for improved oral delivery and photostability of methotrexate. Int J Nanomedicine 2019; 14: 4949-60.
[http://dx.doi.org/10.2147/IJN.S211014] [PMID: 31308665]

[81]   Desai P, Thakkar A, Ann D, Wang J, Prabhu S. Loratadine self-microemulsifying drug delivery systems (SMEDDS) in combination with sulforaphane for the synergistic chemoprevention of pancreatic cancer. Drug Deliv Transl Res 2019; 9(3): 641-51.
[http://dx.doi.org/10.1007/s13346-019-00619-0] [PMID: 30706304]

[82]   Verma R, Kaushik D. Development, Optimization, characterization and impact of *in vitro* lipolysis on drug release of telmisartan loaded SMEDDS. Drug Deliv Lett 2019; 9(4): 330-40.
[http://dx.doi.org/10.2174/2210303109666190614120556]

[83]   Verma R, Kaushik D. Design and optimization of candesartan loaded self-nanoemulsifying drug delivery system for improving its dissolution rate and pharmacodynamic potential 2020.

CHAPTER 2

Introduction to Lipid-Based Drug Delivery Systems for Oral Delivery

Deepak Kaushik[1,*]**, Ravinder Verma**[1]**, Rekha Rao**[2] **and Prerna Kaushik**[1]

[1] *Department of Pharmaceutical Sciences, Maharshi Dayanand University, Rohtak (Haryana), 124001, India*

[2] *Department of Pharmaceutical Sciences, Guru Jambheshwar University, Hisar (Haryana), India*

Abstract: Lipid-based formulations (LBFs) are an alluring alternative among novel drug delivery formulations that are used for the improvement in solubility and bioavailability of drugs that are impossible to dissolve because of their limited solubility in the gastrointestinal tract. As a controlled and targeted formulation, LBDDS includes the discharge of drugs in a controlled manner, high drug loading capacity (as compared to others), biodegradable and biocompatible, carrying capabilities for both lipophilic and hydrophilic drugs and excipients with less risk profile. The most imperative classification in novel drug delivery systems is LBFs including self-emulsifying lipid formulations, lipid solutions and lipid suspensions. Emulsions, microemulsion, nanoemulsion, liposomes, solid lipid nanoparticles, niosomes, liposheres, ethosomes, self-emulsifying drug delivery system and self-microemulsifying drug delivery systems. GI lipid digestion is a mechanism of lipid-based drug delivery systems that is based on the dispersion of oil droplets to give a fine formulation of emulsion, hydrolysis of fatty acid esters with the help of enzymes at the emulsion water interface, desorption and dispersion of insoluble lipid products for absorption. Various mechanisms for upgrading the drug retention include improvement in dissolution/solubilization rate, the extension of gastric retention time; changes in the physical barrier role of the gastrointestinal tract, change in biochemical hindrance capacity of the GI tract, drug assimilation through the intestinal lymphatic system, all of these are discussed in detail. Lipid digestion, hydrophobic nature of the API and mean emulsion droplet sizes are various formulations factors that influence the bioavailability of drugs from LBDDS. Porter outlined seven regulations for the development of LBFs. This chapter highlights various types of lipid-based drug delivery systems with their benefits and drawbacks.

Keywords: Formulation factors, Lipid-based drug delivery systems, Lipid digestion, Mechanisms improving drug retention, Self micro-emulsifying drug delivery system, Solid lipid nanoparticles.

* **Corresponding author Deepak Kaushik:** Department of Pharmaceutical Sciences, Maharshi Dayanand University, Rohtak (Haryana), 124001, India; Tel: +91 9315809626; E-mail: deepkaushik1977@gmail.com

LIPID-BASED DRUG DELIVERY SYSTEM (LBDDS)

These are alluring alternative among novel drug delivery systems that are employed for the enhancement in solubility and bioavailability of drugs that are otherwise impossible to dissolve because of their capacity to maintain the drug solubility in the gastrointestinal tract. Nowadays, roughly 40% of marketed products and over 70% of the pipeline candidates are used as top pharmaceutical administrations containing ineffectively soluble drugs. The predominant therapeutic effectiveness of these inadequately soluble molecules (BCS-II and IV) might be the rationale that they cannot be constantly kept away from drug advancement and optimal formulation methodologies are needed to improve their absorption in the systemic circulation. Although there are traditional methodologies for dealing with poor water solubility, still, novel drug delivery systems (DDS) are necessary for building up a steady and worthy drug formulation. The most imperative classification in novel DDS is lipid-based formulations (LBFs) such as lipid solutions, self-emulsifying lipid formulations and lipid suspensions. The LBFs are frontline formulation innovation to deal with the inadequately aqueous-soluble candidates. The LBFs can be intended to maintain the drug component in the solubilized form and keeping solubilization by avoiding the dissolution step of inadequate water-soluble candidates. These kinds of formulations are recommended for different types of benefits such as lessening the food effect with inter-subject variation, simplicity of formulation designing and the risk of manufacturing and utilizing regular ingredients accessible in the marketplace. In spite of these favorable circumstances, not many items are accessible into the present marketplace, maybe due to constrained information regarding *in vitro* evaluations (for forecasting of *in vivo* fate) and lack of comprehension of biopharmaceutical and pharmacokinetic parts of lipid products after oral ingestion [1].

Poor drug solubility is often experienced issue for pharmaceutical scientists as it influences the drug capacity of a new chemical entity (NCE). Since the vast majority of the NCE prepared, almost (half of them) are hydrophobic. The utilization of LBDDS has turned out to be prevalent for pre-clinical investigations to therapeutic strategies [2].

LBDDS gives a reasonable method for target-specific and additionally time-controlled delivery of drugs. Inadequately water-soluble drugs are extremely challenging to prepare to dosage forms because of their less solubility and subsequently less bioavailability. LBDDS have taken much consideration at present because of their capability to boost the solubility and bioavailability of inadequately water-soluble drugs. Furthermore, the unquestionable focal points are a high level of biocompatibility and versatility [3].

The retention of drugs from LBFs depends on different variables including particle size, emulsification degree, dispersion rate and precipitation of drug upon dispersion. LBFs may include oil solutions or suspensions, emulsions, SMEDDS/SNEDDS. Some of the drugs that are efficiently promoted in the market as LBFs are cyclosporine A, calcitrol, tipranavir, ritonavir [4].

LBDDS includes three elements as features of formulation excipients *i.e.* surfactant, co-surfactant and oil (lipid). It is the one of a kind property of lipids *viz*, their physicochemical assorted variety, biocompatibility and demonstrated capacity to upgrade oral bioavailability of inadequately water-soluble and particular lymphatic take-up of lipophilic drugs that have made them an incredibly alluring applicant as a carrier for oral formulations.

LBFs solubilized in adequate quantities of the drug, enhance scattering of the dosage form in the intestine. When the drug is present in solubilized/dispersed state, it improves and encourages retention of the drug into the intestinal mucosal cells and the systemic circulation [5].

A Perfect Oral Lipid-Based Dosage Forms Must Meet Various Aspects

Following are various aspects that should be followed to obtain lipid-based dosage forms:

1. It ought to solubilize the therapeutic quantities of drugs into dose formulation.
2. It ought to keep up sufficient drug solubility over the whole timeframe of realistic usability of the drug item (by and large two years) under all expected storage circumstances.
3. It ought to give satisfactory chemical and physical stability for the drug and formulation excipients.
4. It must be made up of affirmed ingredients that should be safe.
5. Once ingested, it ought to encourage dispersion of the dosage forms in the intestinal environment and keep up drug solubilization in the dispersed state.
6. It should adjust to the digestion mechanism of the GI tract with the end goal that assimilation either improves or keeps the drug in solubilized form.
7. It should transport the drug into intestinal mucosal cells. So that, drug is retained into the systemic circulation and the cells.

These necessities can make the formulation and assessment of LBFs very difficult. In spite of their significance, an outline of LBFs to address these difficulties is still to a great extent an experimental exercise. This survey will plot a few rules and methodologies in building up these formulations, highlighting the difficulties of every one of these necessities and featuring cases of fruitful LBFs.

Benefits of LBDDS

Their various benefits include:

1. Discharge of drug in a controlled and targeted manner
2. Maintains stability of the product
3. Higher and better drug content
4. The capability of entrapping both lipophilic and hydrophilic drugs
5. Biodegradable and biocompatible in nature
6. Excipients resourcefulness
7. Formulation resourcefulness
8. Less risk profile
9. Passive and non-invasive type of formulation [3].

LIPID FORMULATION CLASSIFICATION SYSTEM

A grouping system for lipid formulations was planned by Pouton in 2000 and modified in 2006. This grouping system distinguishes lipid formulations and offers a rule for contrasting different formulations and information from various laboratories. Lipid formulation classification system was presented by Pouton 2000 that empowers understanding of *ex vivo* studies and helps in recognition of the most fitting formulations for the particular drugs (*i.e.* with indication to their physicochemical characteristics). Table **2** shows the basic contrasts between different types of lipid-based formulations.

This system quickly characterizes LBFs into four types based on composition, feasible impact of dilution and digestion with the capacity to anticipate the drug precipitation. The principle part of the lipid based formulations is to encourage elucidation *in vivo* studies more promptly and distinguishing the most proper formulation for particular drugs with the allusion to their physicochemical characteristics [6 - 8].

Four Types of LFCS

The oil/surfactant mixtures have the capacity to maintain the drug in scattered form into GI media. The formulation adequately consisting of oil are of Type I and the formulation consisting of oil, surfactant and co-surfactant are of Type IV. On the other hand, oil/surfactant mixes, formulating the two transitional types (Type II and III). The Type I, oily formulations don't scatter when they mix up with aqueous media and they must be processed by the GI lipases keeping in mind the end goal to disperse the drug. This type is appropriate for defining exceptionally lipophilic drugs of elevated log P value. Type II and III kind of formulations with oil/surfactant mixtures can self-emulsify when getting in touch with aqueous media. Formulation Type II is comprised of water-insoluble surfactants with HLB <12 that create coarse emulsions when getting in contact with aqueous media. Then again, Type III oil/surfactant preparations comprise of water-soluble type surfactants, HLB >12 delivering finely dispersed nanoemulsion, that is appropriate for preparations of drugs with log P in the vicinity of 2 and 4. Type IV formulations comprise water-soluble surfactants with hydrophilic co-solvents. Their flexibility is the upgraded solvent capability for BCS II drugs that are hydrophobic however not lipophilic (or that consist of less to medium lipophilicity), with the preparation of micellar solutions by solubilized drug on dilution. In any case, expanded extents of hydrophilic surfactants containing PEG chains are required for Type IV systems to cover o/w interface and to give the stearic block to the pancreatic lipase for their activity. In this manner, it suppresses digestion and retention of the drug. Likewise, because of the occurrence of co-solvent into Type IV, their solvent capacity diminishes by scattering in water [9].

Classification System for Lipid Formulations

In 2000, Pouton introduced a lipid formulation classification system and the 'Type' of formulation was introduced in 2006.

Type I – Type I system indicates the weak early dispersion in the aqueous phase and requires digestion by pancreatic lipase/co-lipase for creating more amphiphilic lipidic digestion products that faciliate drug conversion into a colloidal aqueous phase. This is an excellent alternative system for drugs producing satisfactory solubility in oils. For example, valproic acid has been dispensed in soft gelatin capsules with corn oil in the lipidic ingredient.

Type II – These preparations include SEDDS in which self-emulsification is usually attained by using surfactant in amount above 25%. These systems offer the benefits of defeating the slow rate of dissolution, typically examined by solid dosage forms that is explained above. These create higher interfacial areas that permit efficient partitioning of drug into the oil globules and aqueous phase at the target site.

Type III - These are generally known as SMEDDS which are described by the inclusion of hydrophilic surfactant (HLB >12) and co-solvent. These are divided into Type III A and III B formulations. For the identification of more lipophobic systems (Type III B), the quantity of lipophobic surfactants with co-surfactants enhances and the lipidic ingredient quantity decreases. Type III B systems usually attain a larger dispersion rate when contrasted with Type IIIA, the drug precipitation threat on the dispersion of formulation that is superior given less lipidic ingredient.

Table 2. Classification of lipid-based drug delivery systems.

Composition	Type I	Type II	Type III (A)	Type III (B)	Type IV
Glycerides	100%	40-80%	<20%	<20%	-
Surfactants (HLB <12)	-	20-60%	-	-	0-20%
HLB >12	-	-	20-40%	20-50%	20-80%
Hydrophilic co-solvents	-	-	0-40%	20-50%	0-80%
Dispersion behavior	No or limited dispersion due to bile salts in GIT	SEDDS	SMEDDS/ SEDDS	SMEDDS	Micellar solution
Particle size	Coarse	100-250 nm	100-250 nm	50-250 nm	<100 nm
Impact of aqueous dilution	Limited importance	Solvent capability unaffected	Some loss of solvent capability	Phase change and loss of solvent capability	Major phase changes and potential loss of solvent capability
Impact of digestibility	Crucial need	Not crucial but may occur	May be crucial but not be inhibited	Not required	Not required
Advantages	GRAS status, excellent, capsule compatibility	Loss of solvent capacity on dispersion	Clear or almost clear dispersion, drug retention without digestion	Clear dispersion drug retention without digestion	Good solvent capability for drugs, disperse to micellar solution
Disadvantage	Poor solvent capability unless drug is highly lipophilic	Turbid o/w emulsion (0.252μm)	Possible loss of solvent capacity on dispersion, less easily digested	Likely loss of solvent capability on dispersion	Loss of solvent capability on dispersion, may not be digestible
Marketed products	Calcitrol (Rocaltrols), Roche	Cyrlosporin A (Sand-immunes), Novartis	Cyrlosporin A (Neorals), Novartis	Tipranavir (Aptivuss), Boehringer Ingelheim	Ritonavir (Norvirs), Abbott, Amprenavir (Agenerases), GSK

Type IV- These systems usually propose improved drug payloads in contrast to the formulations having simple glycerides lipids and creating very fine dispersion when added in aqueous media. Amprenavir (Agenerase®) is an example of a Type IV formulation that acts as an HIV protease inhibitor in the capsule dosage form. This formulation consists of TGPS, PEG 400 and PG which are used as surfactant, co-surfactant and co-solvent, respectively [10].

APPROACHES IN LBDDS

Many LBFs are available in the pharmaceutical market. Some of the approaches are given in Fig. (**1**).

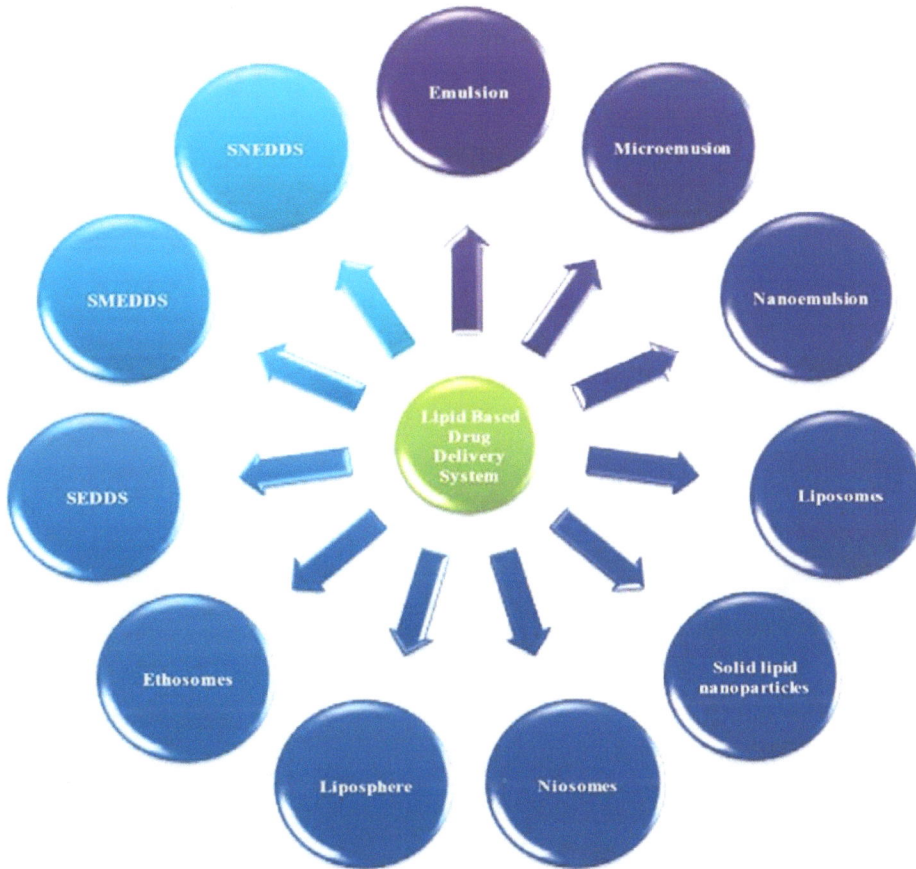

Fig. (1). Various approaches for lipid-based drug delivery systems.

Emulsion

These are a biphasic mixture of two immiscible phases in which a surfactant is incorporated to stabilize the dispersed droplets. An appropriate decision of surfactant and assembling circumstances is essential for the stabilization of the blend [3].

Due to the antibacterial and anti-inflammatory effect of artemisia argyi oil (AAO) is used widely that blocked by its instability with air, light and heat partly. To find out a solution for this, Hu *et al.,* formulated AAO-loaded antibacterial MCs containing Hap/poly(melamine formaldehyde) composite as a pickering emulsifier [11].

Ashara *et al.* developed an emulsion of chloramphenicol that contained parker neem®, peppermint oils, olive and PEG-400 that was safe to use and highly effective than chloramphenicol eye caps [12].

Microemulsion

These are stable systems made up of oil, surfactant/co-surfactant and water, creating a translucent-transparent system whose droplet size lies in micron. Microemulsion can be o/w or w/o in nature relying on the drug being used.

A hydrophobic drug forming an o/w emulsion will transfer from the oil stage to the watery stages relying upon the partition coefficient. The administration route of micro-emulsion can be oral, ocular, pulmonary, nasal, vaginal and intravenous [13].

Soleymani *et al.,* enhanced dermal delivery of finasteride using microemulsion systems with the droplet size range of 5–17 nm and pH rage of 5.1–5.7. From the results, the drug release was 49.5% within 24 hours. These kinds of formulations increased the flux and permeability coefficient from the rat skin. The MEs that exhibit 99.9% drug release after 6 months of stability study [14].

Uchiyama *et al.,* formulated the microemulsion of food-grade with rice glycosphingolipids for increasing the oral absorption of coenzyme Q10 [15].

Zhoua *et al.,* developed microemulsion that contained encapsulated drugs (β-elemene and PTX), mal-DOPE-PEG), thiol conjugated site (maleimide-modified PEGylated 1,2-dioleoyl-sn-glycero-3-phosphoethanolamine, tumor-targeting ligand (3'-end thiolated SYL3C aptamer), pH-sensitive ingredient (DOPE) and other necessary ingredients that helps in the treatment of colon-rectal cancer [16].

Wang *et al.,* developed a eutectic oil-based microemulsion of tacrolimus used in atopic dermatitis that enhanced percutaneous drug delivery and also enhanced the treatment efficacy by decreasing its side effects [17].

Nanoemulsion

These are not formed precipitously; an outer shear must be connected to burst the bigger droplets to littler ones. An extraordinary shear is connected to defeat the impacts of surface pressure to break the droplets into those of nanoscale range.

Nanoemulsions are valuable dispersions of deformable nanoscale droplets with flow characteristics that vary from fluid to exceedingly solid and optical characteristics extending from opaque to transparent. In addition, nanoemulsions are progressively being exploited for commercial use, since they were regularly formulated utilizing altogether less surfactant rather than nanostructured lyotropic microemulsion phases [18].

Jiang *et al.,* developed lactoferrin nanoemulsion loaded HupA for targeted drug transport *via* the intranasal route [19].

Hosny *et al.,* developed saquinavir mesylate nanoemulsion loaded transdermal films [20].

Liposomes

These are vesicular structures, including a phospholipid bilayer encompassing a fluid compartment. Lipophilic drugs can be incorporated into the phospholipid bilayer membrane. Liposomes demonstrate immense potential as an active innovation for upgrading the oral bioavailability of ineffectively soluble drugs, including proteins and peptides. They are utilized as an anti-cancer treatment for focusing on the intense cancer particle to the site of target. This reality can be upheld by huge advancement in immune liposomes (conjugating monoclonal antibodies to liposomes). They are additionally appropriate for the oral inoculation system. Liposomal formulations are regularly viewed as safe because of the GRAS status of the phospholipids ingredients. They are generally utilized as parenteral or injectables (*e.g.* Doxil®) [21, 22].

Akbar *et al.,* developed bombesin receptor-targeted liposomes for enhanced delivery to lung cancer cells. Liposomes produced desirable colloidal characteristics with good stability upon storage. With the help of flow cytometric and microscopic studies, it showed that fluorescently labeled cystabn-decorated liposomes accumulated more extensively in GRPR over-expressing cells than matched liposomes that contain no cystabn targeting motif [23].

Guimaraes *et al.,* investigated the protective effect of freeze-dried liposomes's on saccharides in encapsulating drugs. They concluded that for the cryo/lyoprotection of liposomes with drug molecules a suitable candidate is sucrose that is located in the lipid bilayer [24].

Zappavigna *et al.,* developed liposomes of urotensin-II-targeted as a new formulation for the treatment of prostate and colon cancer cells [25].

Solid Lipid Nanoparticles

These are sub-micron type colloidal carriers going from 50 to 1000 nm that consist of physiological lipids, scattered in aqueous or water surfactant solution. SLNs exhibit exceptional features such as vast surface area, less size, high drug loading and lastly, interaction of phases at the interface are appealing for their ability that increases execution of the formulations. They have stability around 3 years and can be made at an industrial scale. These have been accounted for expanding the bioavailability of a few drugs as reported in the case of cyclosporine A and vinpocetine [26].

Cervantes *et al.,* formulated stearic acid-based SLN with glucocorticoids to protect auditory cells from cisplatin-induced ototoxicity [27].

Essaghraoui *et al.,* developed SLNs to improve topical delivery of cyclosporine A [28].

Niosomes

These are novel drug delivery systems, in which vesicles are used to encapsulate the drug. These vesicles are made up of a bilayer of non-ionic surfactants with the name niosomes. The niosomes comprises of a surfactant bilayer with its hydrophilic ends uncovered outside and hydrophobic chains within the vesicle. The shape and size of niosomes are little and minuscule. Fundamentally like liposomes, they offer a few favorable circumstances over them. Niosomes have been lately appeared to increment transdermal drug delivery significantly and can be utilized as a part of targeted drug delivery and in this way, expanded investigation in these arrangements can give new strategies to drug delivery [29].

Yoshida *et al.,* found that by selecting stable noisome-forming materials such as polyoxyethylenealkylethers, there is the possibility of peroral administration of 9-desglycinamide 8-arginine vasopressin (DGAVP). *In vitro* intestinal assimilation of encapsulated DGAVP into niosomes was carried using an intestinal loop model to simulate an *in vivo* state. The results showed that DGAVP entrapped into niosomes could achieve relatively greater concentrations into the acceptor phase of rat intestinal lumen when compared with a DGAVP solution and DGAVP in presence of empty niosomes after 2 hrs [30].

Machado *et al.* designed niosomes that were encapsulated in biohydrogels based on mixtures of gelatin and kappa-carrageenan (k-carrageenan, k-C) for tunable delivery of phytoalexin resveratrol [31].

Lipospheres

These are lipid-based encapsulation systems, produced for parenteral, oral and topical drug delivery of bioactives. Lipospheres comprise of aqueous dispersible solid miniaturized scale particles that have their diameter between 0.1 to 100 μm. They contain a strong hydrophobic lipidic center (*e.g.* triglycerides) with the help of phospholipids layers implanted on their surface. On the other hand, the inner center containing a pharmaceutical bioactive material dissolved or dispersed in the solid lipid matrix. The liposphere system has been utilized for the controlled discharge of different kinds of drugs together with local anesthetics, antibiotics, anti-inflammatory candidates and anti-cancer candidates. They have likewise been effectively utilized as transporters for vaccines and adjuvants [32].

Kommineni *et al.* developed thymoquinone and cabazitaxel co-loaded lipospheres as a synergistic combination that is an efficient drug delivery vehicle in breast cancer [33].

Esposito *et al.*, developed clotrimazole liposphere gel for the treatment of candidiasis. Leakage tests and adhesion defined its prolonged adhesion, indicating its appropriateness for vaginal application [34].

Singh *et al.*, invented a novel formulation of phospholipid lipospheres with dried rifampicin co-spray for oral delivery [35].

Ethosomes

These are lipidic vesicles that comprise of phospholipids and alcohol (isopropyl alcohol and ethanol) in moderately high concentration with water. These are soft vesicles formulating from ethanol (in higher amounts), phospholipids and water. These may capture drug particles in different physicochemical attributes *i.e.* hydrophobic, lipophobic or amphiphilic. Nano-meter to microns may be the size range of ethosomes. The principal preferred perspective of ethosomes over liposomes is the expanded penetration of the drug. The component of the drug retention from the ethosomal formulations isn't clear. The drug retention most likely occurs in the following two stages: Ethanol impact and Ethosomes impact. Ethosomes have a greater penetration rate through the skin when contrasted with liposomes. Consequently, these can be utilized generally set up of liposomes. Ethosomes have turned into a region of the research area, in light of their upgraded skin penetration, enhanced drug delivery, expanded drug entrapment proficiency and so forth [36].

Shukla *et al.*, designed a topical gel of ethosomes containing melatonin that prevents UV radiation with pseudoplastic rheological behavior, spreadability and optimum pH. It also defined a maximum % *in vitro* drug permeation having flux 13.85 $\mu g/cm^2/hr$ and it followed zero-order release kinetics that was beneficial for topical delivery of a drug [37].

Fu *et al.*, designed a gel formulation of ethosomes that improved the transdermal delivery of thymosin β-4 by the ethanol infusion method [38].

Chandra *et al.*, formulated a gel of ethosomes containing methotrexate with salicylic acid that is used for the cure of psoriasis [39].

Self-emulsifying Drug Delivery System (SEDDS)

SEDDS have improved the bioavailability of the inadequately water-soluble and remarkably penetrable compounds. SEDDS involve a characterized blend of lipidic excipients, including transparent oils, non-ionic surfactants and co-surfactants, which may likewise co-solvents. SEDDS works as transporters for lipophilic drugs having less solubility and henceforth less bioavailability [40].

Upon mild disturbance initiated with dilution in the aqueous phase, for example, GI fluids or distilled water, these systems can result in fine o/w emulsions or microemulsions. These are related to the creation of expansive surface area dispersions that give ideal circumstances to improve retention of inadequately water-soluble drugs [41].

Certain polymers such as natural polymers (guar gum and latex), manufactured polymers (PVP, PVC) can be added into SEDDS to accomplish controlled or sustained discharge of drugs [42].

The GI irritation caused by a drug can be stayed away from or decreased by SEDDS by developing the oily globules subsequently lessening the get in touch time of the drugs with GI tract. The SEDDS blend can be packed either in hard or soft gelatin capsules for the simple delivery of SEDDS formulations [43].

Depending on the size of droplets, the SEDDS can be characterized into two types:

SMEDDS AND SNEDDS

These are an isotropic blend of natural or synthetic oils; surfactants and at least one hydrophilic co-surfactants which upon gentle agitation initiated by dilution in aqueous media, for example, GI liquids can result in fine o/w emulsions or microemulsions. SMEDDS show the formulations developing transparent microemulsion with droplet size below 100 nm. SEFs disperse into the GI tract and the digestive associated movement of the stomach with the intestinal system gives the tumult that is important to self-emulsification.

Fine oil in water droplets would pass quickly from the stomach and furthermore disperse the drug quickly all through the GI tract and limiting the irritation of GIT because of broadened contact between bulk drug candidates and the gut wall. The SMEDDS are physically stable and are anything but difficult to make when contrasted with an emulsion that is sensitive in nature with metastable dispersed forms.

The proficiency of drugs added into SMEDDS formulation is reliant upon the specific physicochemical compatibility of a drug or a drug system. Along these lines, phase diagram and pre-formulation solubility investigations are essential keeping in mind the end goal to get an optimal formulation design. Utilization of systemic strategies such as Design of Experiment (DoE) or quality by design (QbD) can likewise be utilized to assemble data for exact and optimum use of independent factors for accomplishing enhanced solubility and enhanced bioavailability [44].

Liu *et al.*, developed nintedanib loaded SMEDDS for the improvement of drug solubility into a defined physical condition with *in vivo* absorption. The formulation cannot exhibit any obvious cytotoxic effect on caco-2 cells. The rate of drug permeability into these cells was increased by 2.8-times in SMEDDS than the solution of drug. After a study of intestinal perfusion, it was shown that in entire intestine, the permeability of NDNB-SMEDDS was enhanced by 3.0- and 3.2-times into the colon compared with the solution of the drug [45].

Nano Lipid Carriers (NLCs)

These are formulated by the mixing of solid lipids into incompatible oil (also referred to as a "liquid lipid"). Because nanostructures lead to improved release rate and loading capacity, NLC formulations are utilized for various routes of administration, like topical application. In the formulation of NLC, the topical application of prednicarbate results in the higher retention of a drug into a topical layer of the skin than emulsion based formulations. Thus, these formulations are suitable for cosmeceuticals. These are intended to remain in the skin without permeation, thereby reducing their systemic effects.

Kim *et al.*, developed a 20(S)-protopanaxadiol loaded NLC formulation for their topical delivery with the help of Box-Behnken Design, which was able to enhance their topical skin deposition [46].

FORMULATION DEVELOPMENT AND CHARACTERIZATION

Booming LBDDS henceforth necessitates an all encompassing way to deal with the formulations. A methodical clarification of the reason might be accomplished by:

(1) Pre-choosing ingredients for their unsaturated FA make up, melting features, emulsification features, the potential effect on enterocytes based drug transportation, disposition and digestibility.

(2) Performing double screening of the pre-chosen ingredients for drug compatibility, solubility, stability with the rate of dissolution/dispersion characteristics (in biorelevant media) to distinguish at least one reasonable systems for more investigations.

(3) Recognizing the formulation method(s) appropriate for the proposed dosage form.

(4) Verifying the *in vivo* execution of the picked formulation system(s) into a suitable animal model.

(5) For drug loading or dissolution rate of optimized formulation if necessary to pick up the control of polymorphic alterations and oxidation.

Parameters to be Judged for the Development of the Formulation

The most important factors influencing the selection of ingredients for LBFs are the following:

1. Solubility
2. Dispersion
3. Digestion
4. Assimilation

Pouton depicted few parameters that should be considered for choosing a lipidic ingredient which include regulatory concerns, toxicity, irritancy, miscibility, solvent capability, morphology at 25°C, digestibility, self-dispersibility, compatibility, the fate of digested products with capsule shell, chemical stability, purity with the price.

Other than these parameters, lipids have been shown to increase the bioavailability of drugs by other means.

GUIDELINES FOR DESIGNING OF LBFS

It is evident that LBFs will persist to be a vital tool to develop lesser soluble drugs; the development of this type of preparations can be a big challenge. From recent times, Porter outlined seven regulations for the development of LBFs which are summarized below:

(1) It is important to maintain drug solubility in formulation after dispersion and digestion

(2) Features of the colloidal species created after digestion in the GI environment are certainly more significant than features of the preparation itself for enhancement of assimilation

(3) Higher concentrations of lipids (>60%), lesser concentrations of surfactant (<30%) and co-solvent (<10%) usually results in a maximum amount of robust drug that solubilized after dilution

(4) MCT may afford higher drug stability and solubility into formulation. On the other hand, LCT assists more efficient development of lipid colloidal species with bile salts and thus may result in greater bioavailability

(5) After dispersion, SMEDDS preparations offer lesser globule size that relies on the surfactant concentration, while non-digestible surfactants generally offer greater bioavailability

(6) If a combination of surfactants is utilized rather than a single, it may result in more efficient dispersion as occurs in the case of Type IV formulations

(7) Type IV kind of preparations may offer greater drug solubility but must be developed carefully to assure that the drug used in the formulation cannot precipitate after dispersion.

During designing oral LBFs for poorly soluble drugs these guidelines should be kept in mind [3].

FORMULATION FACTORS INFLUENCING BIOAVAILABILITY OF DRUGS FROM LBDDS

Various factors influencing the bioavailability of drugs are discussed below:

Lipid Digestion

If drugs have greater solubility in lipidic vehicles, it can be predicted that it passes through the GIT added into lipid globules demonstrating that the digestion of lipidic ingredient would depend on its gastric emptying rate. Thus, cautious selection of lipidic ingredients can control the assimilation rate of the drug [47].

Mean Droplet Size of Emulsion

According to some researchers, this factor specifies the type and quality of LBDDS. Upon dilution of SEDDS and SMEDDS with aqueous media, the size of droplets of dispersion is primarily affected by the concentration and type of surfactant(s). Higher concentration of surfactant results in the smaller globule size of the emulsion that is responsible for faster drug discharge [48].

Instant creation of emulsion beneficially presents the drug in a dissolved state and results in small globule size which offers a greater interfacial surface area. These kinds of properties result in faster drug discharge from the emulsion in a reproducible manner [6].

The charge on the globules of an emulsion is positive or negative. As the mucosal lining having the negatively charged, a positive charge of emulsion globules can penetrate deeper into the ileum and thus cationic emulsions demonstrate better bioavailability than anionic emulsions [49].

Hydrophobic Nature of API

Highly hydrophobic drugs of log P value >5 can be transported in the lymphatic system with the process of partitioning into chylomicrons and can evade the first-pass metabolism [50].

Chemism of Lipids

The nature of lipids plays a vital role because digestible lipids may influence assimilation to distinguish from that of non-digestible lipids. Improvement in the drug assimilation was reported in LCT contrasted to MCT in SMEDDS. So far, this cannot be considered a rule.

Ingredient Selection for LBFs

Chemically, lipidic ingredients are taken as one of the main ingredient classes available at present. Various subcategories of lipids exist and new lipid-based ingredients enter the market regularly which offer flexibility for choosing an appropriate ingredient for the formulator, but at the same time the formulator should be careful about the selection of specific ingredients [51].

ANALYSIS OF EXCIPIENTS IN LBDDS

Chemical Analysis

The composition of lipidic ingredients such as esters, ethers and distribution of FA can be determined by HPLC and GC techniques. Moisture content must be analyzed for hygroscopic or high HLB value excipients.

Physical Analysis

Lipids have a higher chemical composition and lead to wide melting points as contrasting into a single melting point. An instrument DSC is used for the investigation of thermal performance of ingredients like melting, solid-solid transition temperatures and crystallization. Solid fat substance of the ingredient related to the temperature can be assayed by nuclear magnetic resonance (NMR). XRD can be utilized for the determination of the crystalline nature of a lipidic ingredient [3].

Analysis of Physiological Effects of Ingredients

Oral assimilation has a variety of physiological effects like retarding gastric emptying, secretion of pancreatic juice, stimulation of bile flow, enhancing the membrane lipid fluidity or acting directly upon the enterocytes based drug transportation and disposition, inhibiting efflux transporters like p-glycoprotein (P-gp) *in vitro* models and can be assessed by using liver and intestinal slices.

These effects occurred due to the increase in oral absorption by lipid-based ingredients [52].

MECHANISM OF LIPID-BASED DRUG DELIVERY SYSTEM

There are three steps for GI lipid digestion:

(i) To prepare a fine emulsion, dispersion of fat droplets takes place.

(ii) At the interface of the emulsion, there is an enzymatic hydrolysis of fatty acid esters.

(iii) Dispersion and desorption of insoluble lipid products for succeeding absorption.

These systems may enhance the absorption from the gastrointestinal tract. Lessening of particle size to molecular level facilitates the solubilization process, altering drug uptake, disposition by enterocyte based transport, efflux and increasing medicament transportation into the systemic circulation by the intestinal lymphatic system. Lipophilic drug absorption can occur by the lipids into the portal blood. Triglycerides (TGs) and long-chain (LC) fatty acids (FAs) take part in extending gastric residence time. Although, a high-fat meal raises the level of TG rich lipoproteins that interacts with drug candidates.

The combination of lipoproteins with drug improves the intestinal lymphatic transportation that causes an alteration in drug disposition and also results in pharmacological actions of poorly soluble drugs [53].

MECHANISMS FOLLOWED BY LBDDS FOR UPGRADING THE RETENTION

There are various mechanisms through which upgradation of the retention takes place as shown in Fig. (**2**) and elaborated below:

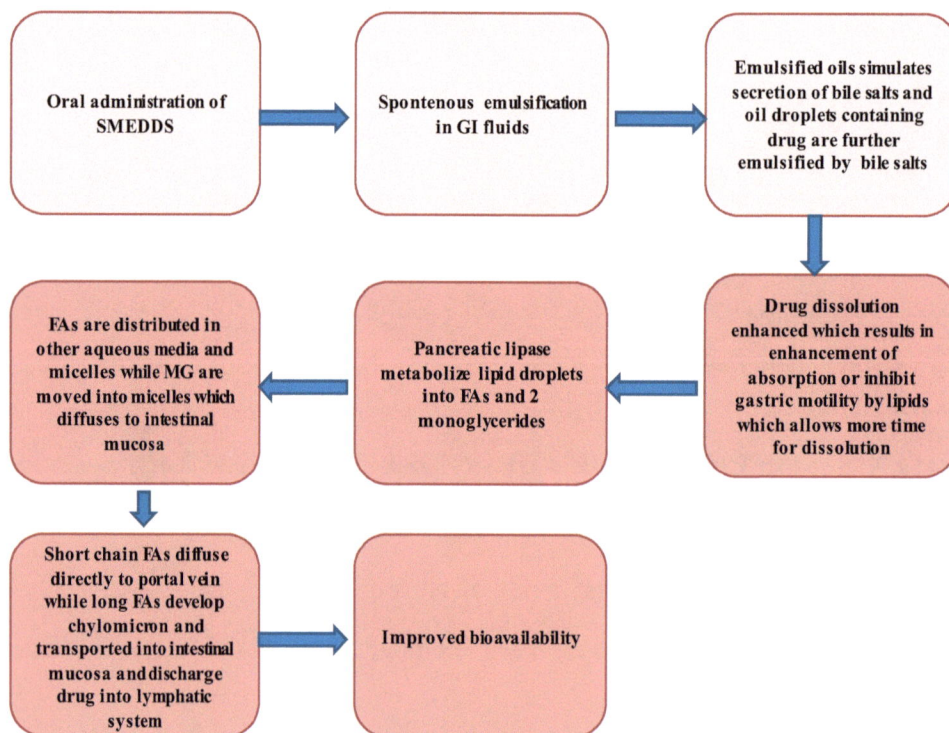

Fig. (2). Mechanism followed by LBDDS for upgrading the retention.

Improved Rate of Dissolution/Solubilization

The occurrence of lipids present in the GI tract initiates gallbladder constrictions, biliary and pancreatic secretions (phospholipids, bile salts and cholesterol) which diminish metabolism and efflux movement. Crude emulsion development advances the solubilization of the co-ingested lipophilic drug because of the development of gastric shear with these items. Lately, it has been discovered that even little quantities of lipid may fortify gallbladder constrictions. Although, the expansion in the biliary secretions, the exogenous lipidic segment of the drug delivery system is subjected to an enzymatic digestion. Esters can be quickly hydrolyzed in presence of the lipolytic products and pancreatic lipase that upon interaction with bile salts/phospholipids leads in the development of various micellar species that anticipate precipitation of the co-ingested lipophilic drug. Exogenous surface-active compounds are included into the delivery system for advanced solubilization of lipophilic candidates [53].

Extension of Gastric Retention Time

Lipids (TGs and long-chain FAs) present in the GI tract slow down the rate of gastric emptying, *i.e.* gastric travel time is upgraded. Accordingly, the retention time of the co-administered lipophilic drug present into small intestine upgrades, that empowers superior dissolution rate of the drug at the site of action and thereby enhances the retention of drug.

Stimulation of Lymphatic Transport

The bioavailability of lipophilic drugs might be improved by initiation of intestinal lymphatic transportation path because of the essence of exceptionally lipophilic drug and its solubility in triglycerides.

Change in the Physical Barrier Role of GI Tract

A variety of lipids has been appeared to modify the physical barrier capacity inside the gut wall due to the improvement of permeability of drugs. For BCS II class candidates, permeability through the GI membrane isn't a constraining advance towards retention. Thus, this process is not believed to be a significant giver for the retention upgrade of lipophilic drugs [54].

Change in Biochemical Hindrance Capacity of GI Tract

Recently, selective surfactants and lipids have been identified to diminish the movement of efflux carrier into the GI wall, bringing about a change in drug retention. In view of the transaction of P-glycoproteins and CYP3A4 movement, the process may lessen intra-enterocyte metabolism too.

Impact of Oils on Retention

These formulations result in a clear o/w emulsion with gentle agitation which might be given by GI movement. SESs additionally enhance the rate of reproducibility of plasma leveltime profile. The impact of lipids upon the bioavailability of orally directed drugs is very confounding because of the different mechanisms by which lipids can modify the biopharmaceutical properties of a drug. They incorporate diminished gastric emptying time, solubility, an expanded dissolution time of drug in the intestinal fluid, development of lipoproteins and advancing the lymphatic transportation of profoundly lipophilic drugs [55].

Digestion of Lipids

On oral intake, the retention of lipid/oil is started into the stomach using gastric lipase (lipid digestion) with the help of lingual lipase into the mouth may increment gastric retention yet SMEDDS formulations are normally filled in hard or soft gelatin capsule. Thus, their substances are discharged in the stomach after the debasement of capsule shell. Emulsification results in retention of lipids in the stomach by the peristaltic movement which is a noteworthy contributing component for the retention of fats. The shear created by peristaltic movement starts the processing by breaking down the formulation into fine emulsion droplets of high surface area. The micro-emulsions formed then enter in the duodenum as tiny lipid droplets and afterwards blend with the bile and the pancreatic juice to experience changes in physical and chemical state.

In the small intestine, the pancreatic lipase collectively with the bile salts and co-lipase, which act on the whole to guarantee the lipid retention and ingestion, finish the breakdown of triglycerides to diglycerides, monoglycerides and unsaturated fats. Elevated concentrations of bile salts have been appeared to hinder pancreatic lipase action in the duodenum. Self-nano/microemulsifying drug delivery systems enhance a drug partitioning rate into aqueous intestinal fluids as well as give steady bioavailability.

Retention of Lipids

The GI tract is lavishly provided with lymphatic as well as blood vessels. In this way, molecules that are assimilated over the small intestinal epithelial cells (enterocytes) can come into any lymphatic system or blood vessels. The dominant parts of consumed substances are transferred in the systematic blood that blood flow rate into the systemic blood is roughly 500-overlap more than the intestinal lymphatic system. Notwithstanding, where the facile diffusion over blood capillary endothelium is constrained, for instance of more molecular weight or colloidal molecules, particular transfer into intestinal lymphatic system may occur since endothelial cells of lymphatics direct that lymphatic vessels which are altogether more permeable than the neighboring blood vessels. Ingestion of macromolecular drug into the oral route and absorption over the enterocyte is restricted and the drug enter the intestinal lymph. It usually occurs because of post-absorptive relationship with colloidal lipoproteins amid transfer over the enterocyte. The small size of lipoproteins manages that diffusion over the vascular endothelium that is constrained by the lymphatic circulation. This process is bolstered by studying lymphatic transportation of transferred DDT, halofantrine and aryl-alkyl hydrocarbons that are solubilised inside a polar lipid center of lymphatic lipoproteins. Lymphatic transportation has been appeared to be a supporter of the oral bioavailability of various lipophilic drugs and different xenobiotics following oral delivery including lipophilic cannabinoids, fat-soluble vitamins and their derivatives, halofantrine, moxidectin, mepitiostane, testosterone analogs, MK386(a5α-reductase inhibitor), penclomedine, naftifine, probucol, CI-976, cyclosporine, ontazolast, retinoids, lycopene, benzopyrene, DDT and analogs, PCBs (polychlorinated biphenyls) plus various lipophilic prodrugs. Conversely, just little amounts of more hydrophilic drugs, for example isoniazid, salicylic acid and caffeine are recouped in lymph following oral delivery [56].

Drug Assimilation through the Intestinal Lymphatic System

Both the lymph and the veins are available into lamina propria, the fundamental intestinal absorptive cells (enterocytes) of the digestive tract. The extent of systematic blood is 500-overlay greater than that of mesenteric lymph and accordingly, most drugs enter into the blood more devotedly than mesenteric lymph. Conversely, following take-up in the enterocytes, unsaturated fatty acids (FAs) and monoglyceride (MG) digestion products are resynthesized to triglyceride (TG) and gathered into colloidal lipoproteins (LPs) inside the endoplasmic reticulum. These LPs are exocytosed over the basolateral layer of the enterocytes and especially get to the mesenteric lymph vessels as their size prohibits simple diffusion over vascular endothelium. Especially, lipophilic drugs (with log P value > 5 and long-chain TG solubility > 50 mg/g) may in this manner get into intestinal lymph through this relationship with LPs in the enterocyte. Fig. (**3**) is demonstrating the digestion and absorption pathway of dietary lipids.

The lipid-based colloidal species are delivered as micelles, blended micelles, vesicles and free unsaturated fats because lipid digestion occurs through facilitated diffusion, passive diffusion and active transportation by enterocyte membrane. Into the cytosol, unsaturated fat-binding protein transfers them from an apical membrane to the endoplasmic reticulum. In this manner, a concentration gradient encourages to take-up FAs in the cells through a transporter interceded route and by interfacing with enterocyte-based carrier and metabolic mechanisms, by this way conceivably changing the drug take-up, aura and the arrangement of metabolites inside enterocyte [57].

Amid the assimilation phase, the drug candidates are normally accessible to the action of cytochrome P450 3A4 (CYP 3A4), introduced at higher concentrations into the erythrocyte situated at the villus tilt in the small intestine of people. These enzymes have importance in expanding the bioavailability of drugs when co-ingested using lipids, which is characteristic of an extra path by which lipids improve oral drug bioavailability.

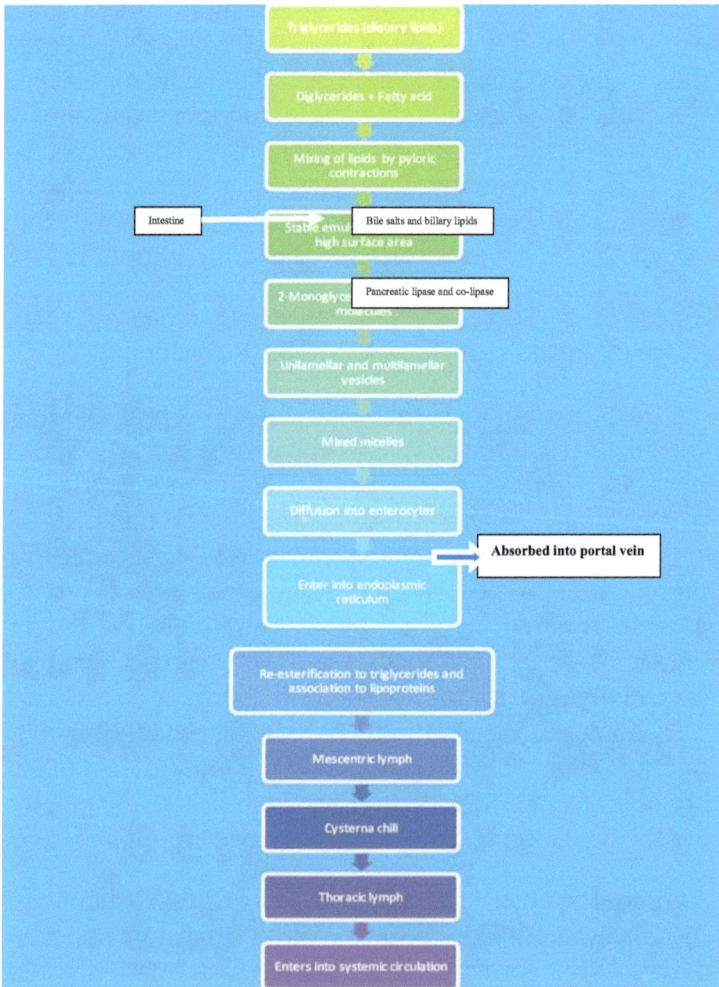

Fig. (3). Schematic representation of the digestion and absorption pattern of dietary lipids.

THERAPEUTIC EQUIVALENCE OF LBDDS

The USFDA esteems medicine formulations helpful in the therapeutic equivalents or pharmaceutical equivalents that have a similar clinical impact and safety profile when directed to patients under the specific conditions in the labeling.

In this background, the U.S. rule is a proof of a bioequivalence or pharmaceutical equivalence that confirms therapeutic equality, thus compatibility.

As indicated by the FDA's Orange Book, pharmaceutically equivalent items ought to contain a similar quantity of active agent in a similar dosage form and have a similar administration route, indistinguishable in concentration or strength and confirms the equal or compendial or other relevant values (*i.e.*, quality, quantity, purity and characteristics). Nonetheless, the Orange Book expresses that pharmaceutically equaivalent items may differ in attributes such as shape, scoring arrangement, discharge rate, bundling, excipients (together with colors, flavors, preservatives), expiry date, within assured restrictions and labeling.

Customarily, qualitative and quantitative correlations of the composition between formulations are the assurance of pharmaceutical equivalence. This strategy might be fitting for simple dosage forms or drug items; an inquiry has been elevated in the matter if it is adequate for complex drug delivery systems, for example, LBFs.

Undoubtedlywith similar qualities depicted by lipid-excipients/surfactants and LBDDS, extra investigation on formulation and potential biopharmaceutical interactions are vital for satisfactory assessment of bioequivalence and pharmaceutical equivalence. A distinction into the preparation of lipid formulation may bring about a major effect on its bioequivalence. This case is shown by using cyclosporine. The generic product of cyclosporine, Sang CyaR oral solution, has less bioavailability than marketed preparation (an oral solution of Neoral IR), when taken with apple juice. It creates the impression that Neoral IR produces a microemulsion while Sang CyaR develops microdispersion after blending with the of apple juice.

Prominently, in any case, the two products were discovered to be bioequivalent, when blended with the help of chocolate milk.

Among, different lipid formulations, the SEDDS offer extra points in terms of greater stability, appropriateness for hydrolytically liable/prone drugs, high drug loading facility, capability for oral drug delivery (solid-SEDDS), simplicity of make up and scale-up if reasonably planned with legitimate choice of ingredients. The novel qualities of lipid excipients and LBDDS have displayed a few difficulties amid the drug advancement and additionally in the foundation of rules and standards. Consideration ought to be given to the unique pharmaceutical features of lipid ingredients and LBDDS. Various investigations are conducted to track the drug solubilization status and investigation of complex associations within the formulation derived from lipids, physiological milieu, surfactant(s) and added drug. The rational design might be accomplished utilizing *in vitro* techniques or additional markers to better predict dynamic alterations of lipidic preparation *in vivo* conditions. The current FDA's activity offers an astounding open door for advancement in regulatory aspects of advanced dosage forms of LBDDS. Great product performance and product quality can be kept up by using the rational design of a lipid-based dosage form [57].

The criteria for the determination of the blend of ingredients for SEDDS formulation ought to incorporate their solubilizing ability with regard to the required dosage of the drug, the capacity to self-emulsification of the system when it comes in contact with GI fluids (by utilization of phase diagram), and their regulatory requirement for for oral administration. The difficulties related to the formulation of SESs include the determination of the right ingredients keeping in view their solvent limit, chemical stability, miscibility, compatibility with capsule shell, regulatory problems, self-dispersibility *etc.* Lipidic ingredients themselves may be subjected to physical alterations or chemical instability after some time, which could conceivably affect drug stability and formulation performance [58].

CONCLUSION

Among the different lipid formulations, the SEDDS offers extra points of interest due to their greater stability, appropriateness for hydrolytically liable/prone drugs, high drug loading facility, capability of oral drug delivery (solid-SEDDS), simplicity of make and scale-up. These novel qualities of lipid excipients and LBDDS have displayed a few difficulties amid the drug advancement and additionally in the foundation of rules and standards. Due consideration ought to be given to the unique pharmaceutical features of lipid ingredients and LBDDS. Various investigations are conducted to track the drug solubilization status and investigation of complex associations with in the formulation derived from lipids, surfactant(s), and added drug into physiological milieu. Rational design of drugs might be accomplished utilizing as a part of *in vitro* techniques or additional markers for the better prediction of dynamic alterations in a lipid formulation *i.e.* *in vivo* condition. The current FDA's policyoffers an amazing open door for upgrading regulatory sciences and fostering advancement in dose forms of LBDDS. Great product performance and product quality can be achieved with the help of the rational design of these formulations.

The criteria for the determination of the blend containing ingredients for SEDDS formulation ought to incorporate their solubilizing ability with regards to the required dosage of medicament, the capacity of self-emulsification of the system when it gets in touch with the GI fluids (with the help of utilization of phase diagram), and their regulatory endorsement state for the oral employment.

The difficulties related to the formulation of SES includethe determination of right ingredients with due thought to their solvent limit, chemical stability, miscibility, compatibility with capsule shell, self-dispersibility, regulatory problems *etc.* Lipidic ingredients themselves may undergo physical alterations or chemical instability after some time, which could conceivably affect medicament stability and formulation performance.

CONSENT FOR PUBLICATION

Not applicable.

CONFLICT OF INTEREST

The author declares no conflict of interest, financial or otherwise.

ACKNOWLEDGEMENTS

Declared none.

REFERENCES

[1]   Tothova Z, Kollipara R, Huntly BJ, *et al.* FoxOs are critical mediators of hematopoietic stem cell resistance to physiologic oxidative stress. Cell 2007; 128(2): 325-39.
[http://dx.doi.org/10.1016/j.cell.2007.01.003] [PMID: 17254970]

[2]   Mahapatra AK, Murthy PN, Swadeep B, Swain RP. Self-emulsifying drug delivery systems (SEDDS): An update from formulation development to therapeutic strategies. Int J Pharm Tech Res 2014; 6(2): 546-68.

[3]   Shrestha H, Bala R, Arora S. Lipid-based drug delivery systems. J Pharm (Cairo) 2014; 2014(1)801820
[PMID: 26556202]

[4]   Kalepu S, Manthina M, Padavala V. Oral lipid-based drug delivery systems–An overview. Acta Pharm Sin B 2013; 3(6): 361-72.
[http://dx.doi.org/10.1016/j.apsb.2013.10.001]

[5]   https://www.europeanpharmaceuticalreview.com/article/49418/lipid-formulations/

[6]   Singh B, Bandopadhyay S, Kapil R, Singh R, Katare OP. Self-emulsifying drug delivery systems (SEDDS): formulation development, characterization and applications. Critic Rev™ in Therapeutic Drug Carrier Sys 2009; 26(5): 24-33.

[7]   Meghani N, Suares D. Self micro-emulsifying drug delivery system (SMEDDS): A promising tool to improve bioavailability. J Pharm Phytother 2013; 2(1): 17-21.

[8]   Porter CJ, Pouton CW, Cuine JF, Charman WN. Enhancing intestinal drug solubilisation using lipid-

based delivery systems. Adv Drug Deliv Rev 2008; 60(6): 673-91.
[http://dx.doi.org/10.1016/j.addr.2007.10.014] [PMID: 18155801]

[9]   Nikolakakis I, Partheniadis I. Self-emulsifying granules and pellets: Composition and formation mechanisms for instant or controlled release. Pharmaceutics 2017; 9(4): 50-8.
[http://dx.doi.org/10.3390/pharmaceutics9040050] [PMID: 29099779]

[10]   Sharma VK, Koka A, Yadav J, Sharma AK, Keservani RK. Self-micro emulsifying drug delivery systems: A strategy to improve oral bioavailability. Ars Pharm 2016; 57(3): 97-109.

[11]   Hu Y, Yang Y, Ning Y, Wang C, Tong Z. Facile preparation of Artemisia argyi oil-loaded antibacterial microcapsules by hydroxyapatite-stabilized Pickering emulsion templating. Colloids Surf B Biointerfaces 2013; 112: 96-102.
[http://dx.doi.org/10.1016/j.colsurfb.2013.08.002] [PMID: 23973909]

[12]   Ashara KC, Shah KV. Emulsion of chloramphenicol: An overwhelming approach for ocular delivery. Folia Med (Plovdiv) 2017; 59(1): 23-30.
[http://dx.doi.org/10.1515/folmed-2017-0007] [PMID: 28384103]

[13]   Muzaffar FA, Singh UK, Chauhan L. Review on microemulsion as futuristic drug delivery. Int J Pharm Pharm Sci 2013; 5(3): 39-53.

[14]   Mohammad Soleymani S, Salimi A. Enhancement of dermal delivery of finasteride using microemulsion systems. Adv Pharm Bull 2019; 9(4): 584-92.
[http://dx.doi.org/10.15171/apb.2019.067] [PMID: 31857962]

[15]   Uchiyama H, Chae J, Kadota K, Tozuka Y. Formation of food grade microemulsion with rice glycosphingolipids to enhance the oral absorption of coenzyme Q10. Foods 2019; 8(10): 502.
[http://dx.doi.org/10.3390/foods8100502] [PMID: 31618946]

[16]   Zhou X, Cao C, Li N, Yuan S. SYL3C aptamer-anchored microemulsion co-loading β-elemene and PTX enhances the treatment of colorectal cancer. Drug Deliv 2019; 26(1): 886-97.
[http://dx.doi.org/10.1080/10717544.2019.1660733] [PMID: 31524012]

[17]   Wang Y, Cao S, Yu K, *et al.* Integrating tacrolimus into eutectic oil-based microemulsion for atopic dermatitis: simultaneously enhancing percutaneous delivery and treatment efficacy with relieving side effects. Int J Nanomedicine 2019; 14: 5849-63.
[http://dx.doi.org/10.2147/IJN.S212260] [PMID: 31440050]

[18]   Kotta S, Khan AW, Ansari SH, Sharma RK, Ali J. Anti HIV nanoemulsion formulation: optimization and *in vitro-in vivo* evaluation. Int J Pharm 2014; 462(1-2): 129-34.
[http://dx.doi.org/10.1016/j.ijpharm.2013.12.038] [PMID: 24374067]

[19]   Jiang Y, Liu C, Zhai W, Zhuang N, Han T, Ding Z. The Optimization design of lactoferrin loaded HupA nanoemulsion for targeted drug transport *via* intranasal route. Int J Nanomedicine 2019; 14: 9217-34.
[http://dx.doi.org/10.2147/IJN.S214657] [PMID: 31819426]

[20]   Hosny KM. Development Of saquinavir mesylate nanoemulsion-loaded transdermal films: Two-step optimization of permeation parameters, characterization and *ex vivo* and *in vivo* evaluation. Int J Nanomedicine 2019; 14: 8589-601.
[http://dx.doi.org/10.2147/IJN.S230747] [PMID: 31802871]

[21]   Laouini A, Jaafar-Maalej C, Limayem-Blouza I, Sfar S, Charcosset C, Fessi H. Preparation, characterization and applications of liposomes: state of the art. J Colloid Sci Biotech 2012; 1(2): 147-68.
[http://dx.doi.org/10.1166/jcsb.2012.1020]

[22]   Wang Q, He L, Fan D, Liang W, Fang J. Improving the anti-inflammatory efficacy of dexamethasone in the treatment of rheumatoid arthritis with polymerized stealth liposomes as a delivery vehicle. J Mater Chem B Mater Biol Med 2020; 8(9): 1841-51.
[http://dx.doi.org/10.1039/C9TB02538C] [PMID: 32016224]

[23]   Akbar MJ, Lukasewicz Ferreira PC, Giorgetti M, Stokes L, Morris CJ. Bombesin receptor-targeted liposomes for enhanced delivery to lung cancer cells. Beilstein J Nanotechnol 2019; 10: 2553-62.
        [http://dx.doi.org/10.3762/bjnano.10.246] [PMID: 31921534]

[24]   Guimarães D, Noro J, Silva C, Cavaco-Paulo A, Nogueira E. Protective effect of saccharides on freeze-dried liposomes encapsulating drugs. Front Bioeng Biotechnol 2019; 7: 424.
        [http://dx.doi.org/10.3389/fbioe.2019.00424] [PMID: 31921827]

[25]   Zappavigna S, Abate M, Cossu AM, *et al.* Urotensin-II-Targeted liposomes as a new drug delivery system towards prostate and colon cancer cells. J Oncol 2019; 20199293560
        [http://dx.doi.org/10.1155/2019/9293560] [PMID: 31929800]

[26]   Garud A, Singh D, Garud N. Solid lipid nanoparticles (SLN): Method, characterization and applications. Int J Curr Pharm 2012; 1(11): 384-93.
        [http://dx.doi.org/10.3329/icpj.v1i11.12065]

[27]   Cervantes B, Arana L, Murillo-Cuesta S, Bruno M, Alkorta I, Varela-Nieto I. Solid Lipid nanoparticles loaded with glucocorticoids protect auditory cells from cisplatin-induced ototoxicity. J Clin Med 2019; 8(9): 1464.
        [http://dx.doi.org/10.3390/jcm8091464] [PMID: 31540035]

[28]   Essaghraoui A, Belfkira A, Hamdaoui B, Nunes C, Lima SAC, Reis S. Improved dermal delivery of cyclosporine A loaded in solid lipid nanoparticles. Nanomaterials (Basel) 2019; 9(9): 1204.
        [http://dx.doi.org/10.3390/nano9091204] [PMID: 31461853]

[29]   Makeshwar KB, Wasankar SR. Niosome: A novel drug delivery system. Asian J Pharm Res 2013; 3(1): 16-20.

[30]   Machado ND, Fernandez MA, Haring M, Sald S, D'ıaz D. Niosomes encapsulated in biohydrogels for tunable delivery of phytoalexin resveratrol. RSC Advances 2019; 9: 7601-9.
        [http://dx.doi.org/10.1039/C8RA09655D]

[31]   Yoshida H, Lehr CM, Kok W, Junginger HE, Verhoef JC, Bouwstra JA. Niosomes for oral delivery of peptide drugs. J Control Release 1992; 21: 145-53.
        [http://dx.doi.org/10.1016/0168-3659(92)90016-K]

[32]   Satheeshbabu N, Gowthamarajan K. Manufacturing techniques of lipospheres: Overview. Int J Pharm Pharm Sci 2011; 3(4): 17-21.

[33]   Kommineni N, Saka R, Bulbake U, Khan W. Cabazitaxel and thymoquinone co-loaded lipospheres as a synergistic combination for breast cancer. Chem Phys Lipids 2019; 224104707
        [http://dx.doi.org/10.1016/j.chemphyslip.2018.11.009] [PMID: 30521787]

[34]   Esposito E, Sguizzato M, Bories C, Nastruzzi C, Cortesi R. production and characterization of a clotrimazole liposphere gel for candidiasis treatment. Polymers (Basel) 2018; 10(2)E160
        [http://dx.doi.org/10.3390/polym10020160] [PMID: 30966196]

[35]   Singh C, Koduri LV, Bhatt TD, *et al.* *In vitro in vivo* evaluation of novel co-spray dried rifampicin phospholipid lipospheres for oral delivery. AAPS PharmSciTech 2017; 18(1): 138-46.
        [http://dx.doi.org/10.1208/s12249-016-0491-5] [PMID: 26902373]

[36]   Parashar T, Sachan R, Singh V, *et al.* Ethosomes: A recent vesicle of transdermal drug delivery system. Int J Res Dev Pharm Life Sci 2013; 2(2): 285-92.

[37]   Shukla R, Tiwari G, Tiwari R, Rai AK. Formulation and evaluation of the topical ethosomal gel of melatonin to prevent UV radiation. J Cosmet Dermatol 2019; 12 Epub ahead of print
        [http://dx.doi.org/10.1111/jocd.13251] [PMID: 31829513]

[38]   Fu X, Shi Y, Wang H, *et al.* Ethosomal gel for improving transdermal delivery of thymosin β-4 2019.
        [http://dx.doi.org/10.2147/IJN.S228863]

[39]   Chandra A, Aggarwal G, Manchanda S, Narula A. Development of topical gel of methotrexate incorporated ethosomes and salicylic acid for the treatment of psoriasis. Pharm Nanotechnol 2019;

7(5): 362-74.
[http://dx.doi.org/10.2174/2211738507666190906123643] [PMID: 31490769]

[40]   Mistry RB, Sheth NS. A review: Self-emulsifying drug delivery system. Int J Pharm Pharm Sci 2011; 3(2): 23-8.

[41]   Gursoy RN, Benita S. Self-emulsifying drug delivery systems (SEDDS) for improved oral delivery of lipophilic drugs. Biomed Pharmacother 2004; 58(3): 173-82.
[http://dx.doi.org/10.1016/j.biopha.2004.02.001] [PMID: 15082340]

[42]   Gajera KG, Raval AG. Formulation and evaluation of orodispersible tablets of paliperidon E. Int J Pharm and Biological Sci Archive 2019; 7(2): 24-36.
[http://dx.doi.org/10.32553/ijpba.v7i2.116]

[43]   Gupta S, Kesarla R, Omri A. Formulation strategies to improve the bioavailability of poorly absorbed drugs with special emphasis on self-emulsifying systems. ISRN Pharm 2013; 2013(4)848043
[http://dx.doi.org/10.1155/2013/848043] [PMID: 24459591]

[44]   Verma R, Kaushik D. Design and optimization of candesartan loaded self-nanoemulsifying drug delivery system for improving its dissolution rate and pharmacodynamic potential 2020.

[45]   Liu H, Mei J, Xu Y, *et al.* Improving The oral absorption of nintedanib by a self-microemulsion drug delivery system: Preparation and *in vitro/in vivo* evaluation. Int J Nanomedicine 2019; 14: 8739-51.
[http://dx.doi.org/10.2147/IJN.S224044] [PMID: 31806968]

[46]   Kim MH, Kim KT, Sohn SY, *et al.* Formulation and evaluation of nanostructured lipid carriers (NLCs) of 20(s)-protopanaxadiol (PPD) by box-behnken design. Int J Nanomedicine 2019; 14: 8509-20.
[http://dx.doi.org/10.2147/IJN.S215835] [PMID: 31749618]

[47]   Nanjwade BK, Patel DJ, Udhani RA, Manvi FV. Functions of lipids for enhancement of oral bioavailability of poorly water-soluble drugs. Sci Pharm 2011; 79(4): 705-27.
[http://dx.doi.org/10.3797/scipharm.1105-09] [PMID: 22145101]

[48]   Tarr BD, Yalkowsky SH. Enhanced intestinal absorption of cyclosporine in rats through the reduction of emulsion droplet size. Pharm Res 1989; 6(1): 40-3.
[http://dx.doi.org/10.1023/A:1015843517762] [PMID: 2717516]

[49]   Čerpnjak K, Zvonar A, Gašperlin M, Vrečer F. Lipid-based systems as a promising approach for enhancing the bioavailability of poorly water-soluble drugs. Acta Pharm 2013; 63(4): 427-45.
[http://dx.doi.org/10.2478/acph-2013-0040] [PMID: 24451070]

[50]   Lin JH, Chen W, King J. The effect of dosage form on oral absorption of L-365, 260, a potent CCK receptor antagonist in dogs. Pharm Res 1991; 8(2): 272-88.

[51]   Khoo SM, Humberstone AJ, Porter CJ, Edwards GA, Charman WN. Formulation design and bioavailability assessment of lipidic self-emulsifying formulations of halofantrine. Int J Pharm 1998; 167(1-2): 155-64.
[http://dx.doi.org/10.1016/S0378-5173(98)00054-4]

[52]   Lalwani JT, Thakkar VT, Patel HV. Enhancement of solubility and oral bioavailability of ezetimibe by a novel solid self nano-emulsifying drug delivery system (SNEDDS). Int J Pharm Pharm Sci 2013; 5(3): 513-22.

[53]   Midha K, Nagpal M, Singh G, Aggarwal G. Prospectives of solid self-microemulsifying systems in novel drug delivery. Curr Drug Deliv 2017; 14(8): 1078-96.
[http://dx.doi.org/10.2174/1567201813666160824123504] [PMID: 27557673]

[54]   Potphode VR, Deshmukh AS, Mahajan VR. Self-micro emulsifying drug delivery system: An approach for enhancement of bioavailability of poorly water-soluble drugs. Asian J Pharm Tech 2016; 6(3): 159-68.
[http://dx.doi.org/10.5958/2231-5713.2016.00023.4]

[55]   Dahan A, Hoffman A. Rationalizing the selection of oral lipid based drug delivery systems by an *in vitro* dynamic lipolysis model for improved oral bioavailability of poorly water soluble drugs. J Control Release 2008; 129(1): 1-10.
[http://dx.doi.org/10.1016/j.jconrel.2008.03.021] [PMID: 18499294]

[56]   Trevaskis NL, Charman WN, Porter CJ. Lipid-based delivery systems and intestinal lymphatic drug transport: a mechanistic update. Adv Drug Deliv Rev 2008; 60(6): 702-16.
[http://dx.doi.org/10.1016/j.addr.2007.09.007] [PMID: 18155316]

[57]   Verma R, Kaushik D. *In vitro* lipolysis as a tool for establishment of IVIVC for lipid based drug delivery systems. Curr Drug Deliv 2019; 16(8): 688-97.
[http://dx.doi.org/10.2174/1567201816666190620115716] [PMID: 31250755]

[58]   Chen ML. Lipid excipients and delivery systems for pharmaceutical development: a regulatory perspective. Adv Drug Deliv Rev 2008; 60(6): 768-77.
[http://dx.doi.org/10.1016/j.addr.2007.09.010] [PMID: 18077051]

CHAPTER 3

Self-Micro Emulsifying Drug Delivery Systems and their Applications

Deepak Kaushik[1,*], Ravinder Verma[1] and Parijat Pandey[2]

[1] *Department of Pharmaceutical Sciences, Maharshi Dayanand University, Rohtak (Haryana), 124001, India*

[2] *Shri Baba Mastnath Institute of Pharmaceutical Sciences and Research, Baba Mastnath University, Rohtak (Haryana), 124001, India*

Abstract: SMEDDS (Type III B systems) are isotropic mixtures of oils, surfactants, co-solvents and co-surfactants that have the capability to create fine o/w microemulsions upon mild stirring followed by dilution in the aqueous phase. They have captured due attention because of their high transparency, high solubilization capacity, thermodynamic stability and simple production method. They also improve oral assimilation and eradicate food effects. There has been an upheaval over the most recent two decades in the usage of microemulsion systems in an assortment of pharmaceutical, chemical and industrial processes. The use of self-microemulsion in pharmaceuticals, as cosmetics agents, for analytical purposes, in biotechnology, as enzymatic reactions, for immobilization of protein, bioseparations and chemical sensor have been described briefly. Oral, topical, parenteral, oculars and pulmonary deliveries are the general routes of drug administration for LBDDS that are discussed in detail. The oral route includes SE capsule, SE sustained/controlled release tablet/capsule/ pellets, SE solid dispersions. This chapter highlights various benefits, drawbacks, selection of ingredients and the applications of self-emulsification in various fields such as cosmetics, analysis, bioseparation and so on.

Keywords: BCS class, Bioseparations by microemulsion, Marketed lipid formulations, SMEDDS, SE capsule, SE pellet.

LIPID-BASED DRUG DELIVERY SYSTEMS

Different formulation techniques can develop lipid-based dosage forms such as solid lipid nanoparticles (SLNs), solid dispersions, self-microemulsifying drug delivery systems (SMEDDS), liposomes and super-saturable self-emulsifying systems. Both lipids (in the form of solid or liquid) and excipients (surfactants,

---

* **Corresponding author Deepak Kaushik:** Department of Pharmaceutical Sciences, Maharshi Dayanand University, Rohtak (Haryana), 124001, India; Tel: +91 9315809626; E-mail: deepakkaushik1977@gmail.com

co-surfactants and co-solvents) are utilized in their formulation not only to improve the bioavailability of the drug but also to assist in the bypass of the erratic assimilation. In addition, lipids and its excipients are known for maintaining the drug in the solubilized form, promoting lymphatic transport, altering epithelium permeability, altering enterocyte based drug transport and inhibiting the p-gp (permeability glycoprotein) efflux [1].

During the last decade, the lipid-based formulation has gained more attention with particular emphasis on SMEDDS because of their less droplet size and high thermodynamic stability [2]. Their emulsions can be o/w, w/o or multiple emulsions [3].

SELF-MICRO EMULSIFYING DRUG DELIVERY SYSTEM

These (Type III B) are isotropic mixtures of oils, surfactants, co-solvents and co-surfactants that have the ability to create fine o/w microemulsions upon mild stirring followed by dilution in the aqueous phase. They disperse quickly in the GI tract due to the peristaltic movement of the stomach and the intestine. They contain a massive amount of co-surfactants but contain less oil quantity that result in higher risk of precipitation of drug. They have gained more attention because of their high transparency, high solubilization capacity, thermodynamic stability and simple production method. They also improve oral assimilation and eradicate the food effects. The diffusion of the drug from oil droplets is the rate-limiting step for dissolution of the drug from SMEDDS, which depends on the surfactant concentration and co-surfactant in the system [4]. Some authors refer self-nanoemulsifying drug delivery systems (SNEDDS) to Type IIIB formulations, which form transparent o/w emulsion of droplets of size less than 100 nm after dilution with distilled water. Most of the marketed lipid formulations belong to Type III [5]. Differences among SEDDS, SMEDDS and SNEDDS are shown in Tables **1** and **2**.

Table 1. Features of SEDDS, SMEDDS and SNEDDS [7].

System/ Characteristic	SEDDS	SMEDDS	SNEDDS
Composition	Simple binary preparations with drug and lipidic ingredients with self-emulsification feature when they come in contact with GI fluids	Consist of drug molecule, oils, surfactant, co-surfactant and co-solvent if required	Consist of drug molecule, oils, surfactant/co-surfactant and co-solvents
Globule size	From 250 nm to 5 μm	100-250 nm	< 100 nm
Appearance	Turbid	Transparent to translucent	Transparent

System/ Characteristic	SEDDS	SMEDDS	SNEDDS
Stability of dispersions	Thermodynamically unstable	Thermodynamically stable	Thermodynamically and kinetically stable
Formulation technique	Their development/optimization may require the development of ternary phase diagrams	For optimization of SMEDDS, Pseudo-ternary phase diagrams are required and the order of mixing preselected components is not important	Techniques for their preparation are not defined clearly, but the order of mixing preselected ingredients is defined

History of Micro-emulsions

T. P.Hoar proposed the term microemulsion (ME). In 1943, Shulman gave alternative names for these systems like transparent emulsion, micellar solution, swollen micelle and solubilized oil. These are created due to the below mentioned properties:

i. Very low level of interfacial tension at the interface of oil/water due to the presence of co-surfactant.
ii. The interfacial layer should be highly flexible and fluid. These two requirements are commonly provided by the selection of appropriate ingredients and their proportions. These conditions result in a thermodynamically optimized formulation that is more stable than traditional emulsions and does not need high energy input for their creation. MEs are clear and their structure cannot be seen through a microscope because of the much smaller size of the particles [6].

Table 2. Comparison between SEDDS and SMEDDS.

SEDDS	SMEDDS
The formulation can be binary with drug and lipidic surfactant and oil	This formulation consists of the drug, surfactant, co-surfactant and oil
Droplet size is between 200 nm-50μm in dispersion and provides more surface area	Droplet size is less than 200 nm in dispersion and provides less surface area
Turbid appearance	Optically transparent to translucent appearance
Thermodynamically unstable in physiological fluids or water	Thermodynamically stable in physiological fluids or water
A ternary phase diagram is required for optimization	A pseudo-ternary phase diagram is required for optimization
Oil concentration in the range of 40-80%	Oil concentration of less than 20%

(Table 2) cont.....

SEDDS	SMEDDS
HLB value of surfactant used <12	HLB value of surfactant used >12

Benefits

Their major benefits include enhancement of oral bioavailability that enables dose reduction, more consistent drug assimilation, selective targeting of drug(s), protection of drug(s) in the gut from its antagonistic environment, controlled delivery profiles, decreased variability, including food effects, protection of susceptible drugs, high drug loading capacity, can be formulated into liquid/solid dosage form, simplicity of production and scale-up [8 - 13].

Drawbacks

The major drawbacks include:

1. Lack of useful predictive *in vitro* models.
2. Conventional dissolution method cannot be used.
3. *In vitro* model requires further development and validation prior to the assessment of its strength.
4. Various prototypes of LBFs requires to be designed and *in vivo* evaluation.
5. The chemical instability of drugs and high concentration of surfactant irritate GIT.
6. Volatile co-solvents are known to migrate into shells of capsules that result in precipitation of hydrophobic drugs.
7. Formulations that contain various ingredients become more challenging to validate [14 - 19].

Formulation

The following points should be taken into account during formulation development of a SMEDDS:

Finding Solubility of the Drug in Various Ingredients

To find out the solubility of the drug, incorporate an excessive amount of drug in the vials, which contains each category ingredients separately. Mix the drug with a glass rod for half-hour and then keep the vials in an ultrasonicator for about 2 hours. Close the vials strongly with a stopper and continuously stir it for three days in an orbital shaker incubator at 25˚C. Then, centrifuge the content of vials at 3500 rpm for 20 min. Take 1 ml of separated supernatants and dissolve in a suitable solvent and analyze for drug content by UV or HPLC analysis. Choose two excipients from each category of ingredients based on the solubility of the drug [20].

Selection of Ingredients

For choosing, the best combination of surfactant and oil, self-emulsification capacity of surfactants with oils is investigated by preparing 10% w/w aqueous solution of each in distilled water. 10 ml solution of each surfactant is used to titrate with each of oil. Record the quantity of oil where turbidity occurs in the emulsion. The combination of oil and surfactant which offers the greatest amount of oil emulsification is chosen.

For choosing co-surfactant, each of them is mixed with chosen surfactant in 1:1 (Smix) and different formulations are formulated with chosen Smix and oil where the concentration of oil ranges from 10-90%. Each formulation (1 g) is mixed with 500 ml of distilled water and clearness of resultant emulsion is noted. Microemulsion region is confirmed by transparent/bluish appearance and macroemulsion area is confirmed by turbid appearance. Co-surfactant that illustrates a higher microemulsion region is chosen [21].

Construction of Ternary Phase Diagram

These are plotted to get the ratios of ingredients that can affect the outcome in maximum ME existence region, as shown in Fig. (**1**). These are plotted with oil, Smix and water employing water titration/water dilution method. In this, different ratios of surfactant:co-surfactant by weight such as 1:1, 1:2, 2:1, 3:1, 3:1 are formulated, vortexed for 5 minutes and kept at 50°C for 1 hrs to achieve an isotropic mixture. These solutions are utilized for developing a mixture that contains oil and Smix in ratios 1:9, 2:8, 3:7, 4:6, 5:5, 6:4,7:3, 8:2, 9:1 and after their preparation, these are vortexed for 5 minutes and kept in the oven at 50°C for 1 hr [22].

Water addition is done gradually and after each addition, the mixtures are visualized for their transparency (turbid or transparent). Turbid samples indicate a coarse emulsion production, whereas a clear isotropic solution shows the production of a ME. The development of microemulsion regions is monitored visually for turbidity–transparency–turbidity [23, 24]. "Chemix® (Arne Standnes), sigma plot® (Systat Software Inc), Design Expert® (state ease), chemdraw® (Cambridge Soft Corporation)" are different software that is utilized to plot the phase diagram [25].

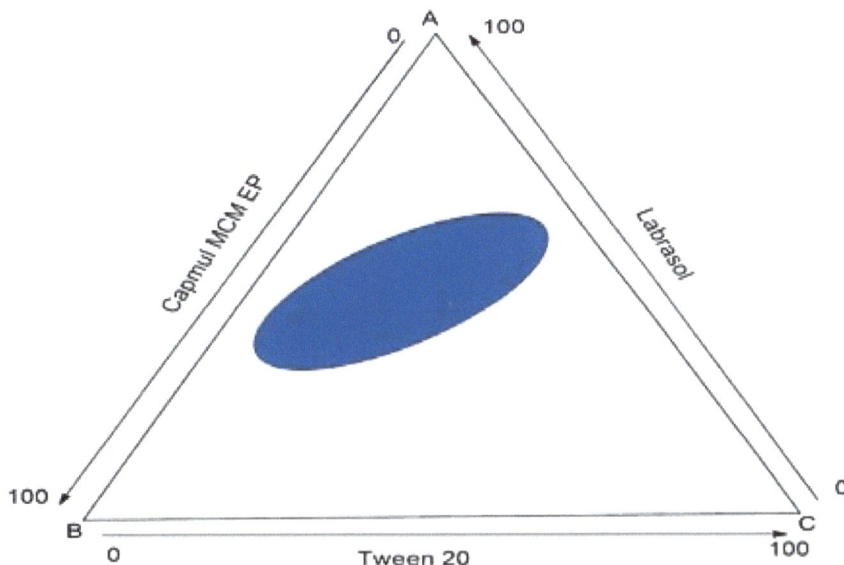

Fig. (1). Pseudo ternary phase diagram showing the microemulsion region in the blue area.

Preparation and Evaluation

From this diagram, concentration and the ratio of ingredients are optimized. By varying the ratio of oil and Smix, various preparations are formulated with and without drug and blended to get an isotropic mixture. Then, these formulations are assessed for various parameters such as globule size, zeta potential, drug assay, % transmittance, % drug discharge, content uniformity and stability, *etc* [26].

Selection of Appropriate Medicament Candidate

Drugs having high doses are not good candidates for these formulations. The solubility of drug and polarity of lipidic ingredients are also key factors for the selection of drug. The polarity relies on HLB value, the unsaturation of the FA and chain length. Maintenance of drug solubility within the GIT is the major hurdle for developing orally administered dosage forms. For hydrophobic molecules that show dissolution-rate-limited assimilation, they enhance the rate and extent of assimilation that result in reproducible blood-time profiles [27].

Lipinski's rule of five is helpful, especially at the early screening phase. It is considered that the rule of five only holds for candidates that are not substrates for active transporters and with growing facts that most drugs are substrates for some efflux or uptake transporters, this limitation must be noted. Log P value alone is unlikely to be enough for identification of the appropriateness of drug for the LBF approach because they do not sufficiently guess latent *in vivo* response [5].

These systems can help out to solve issues of all categories of BCS class drugs as represented in Table **3**.

Table 3. Applications of SMEDDS in different BCS class drugs.

BCS Class	Problems	Absorption	Solubility	Permeability	Examples
I	Enzymatic degradation, gut wall efflux	Well absorbed	High	High	Metoprolol, diltiazem, propranolol
II	Solubilization and bioavailability	Well absorbed	Low	High	Telmisartan, rosuvastatin, candesartan
III	Enzymatic degradation, gut wall efflux and bioavailability	Variable	High	Low	Cimetidine, acyclovir, captopril
IV	Solubilization, enzymatic degradation, gut wall efflux	Poorly absorbed	Low	Low	Hydrochlorothiazide, taxol, furosemide

Role of SMEDDS for BCS Class Drugs

BCS is a logical classification of a drug candidate in scrutiny of its aqueous solubility and permeability associated with *in vitro* and *in vivo* bioavailability of drugs. At the point when joined with *in vitro* dissolution features of the drug items, BCS judges two central points: solubility and intestinal permeability, which represent the extent and degree of oral drug retention from solid dosage formulations and, eventually, its systemic retention. Because of this reason, it is an essential parameter in drug development, particularly in the advancement of oral drug products.

The Food and Drug Administration (FDA) measures for solubility grouping of a drug in BCS depends on the highest dose strength in immediate-release (IR) oral product. A drug is considered exceedingly soluble when the highest strength is soluble in 250 ml (this volume is obtained from normal bioequivalence studies). If it does not solubilize, then the drug compound is considered to be inadequately soluble. Then again, permeability characterization is constructed particularly relating to the degree of intestinal ingestion of a drug compound over the intestine of humans or in creatures or *in vivo* models. Drug molecule is considered permeable when the degree of intestinal retention is calculated 90% or higher in light of mass-adjust or judging against *i/v* reference dose. The bioavailability of BCS II class drugs is probably dissolution rate constrained. BCS class II drugs have been on focused for solubility improvement and a few formulation strategies have been developed for these. In case of BCS class III drugs, the bioavailability is permeability rate constrained, however dissolution is probably going to happen swiftly. Along these lines for class III drugs, preparing IR solid dosage products with retention enhancers can be a reasonable choice to boost their permeability. In the case of BCS IV class drugs, bioavailability is constrained by both the rate of dissolution and the intestinal permeability. Due to less permeability of this class, drugs have poor possibility for formulation development since solubility and rate of dissolution alone would not facilitate their bioavailability. In any case, these classes of candidates can not be disregarded in light of their permeability problems. Along these lines, the existing methodologies being employed for BCS class II drugs, jointly with retention enhancers, can be connected to prepare class IV candidates.

SMEDDS and their potential to solve various issues associated with the drug molecule class I drugs that are water-soluble and permeable to the GI tract. This class does not experience the ill effects of retention or permeation issues that can influence oral drug bioavailability. While classes II, III and IV have drugs facing issues in solubility and permeability and the bioavailability in the systemic circulation after the drug is taken orally. Class II, III and IV form around 80% of the drugs accessible in the marketplace.

Mechanism of Self-emulsification

Self-emulsification exists when the entropy change is higher than the energy necessary to expand the surface area. In case of SMEDDS, free energy of the creation of globules is very low (positive or even negative) that consequences in spontaneous emulsification. For the existence of emulsification, there must be no resistance against surface shearing for the interfacial structure that occurs between the oil and aqueous continuous phases, which is created upon the incorporation of a binary mixture (oil/non-ionic surfactant) to water. This is followed by solubilization within the oil phase, as the effect of aqueous penetration through the interface. Aqueous penetration will result in the development of the dispersed liquid crystal (LC) phase.

So, after gentle agitation of SMEDDS, water quickly penetrates the aqueous cores and leads to interface disruption and development of globules. This LC phase is liable for the high stability of the resultant ME against coalescence [28 - 36].

APPLICATIONS OF SMEDDS

For more than the last two decades, MEs are used in various pharmaceutical, chemical, industrial processes and so on, as shown in Fig. (2).

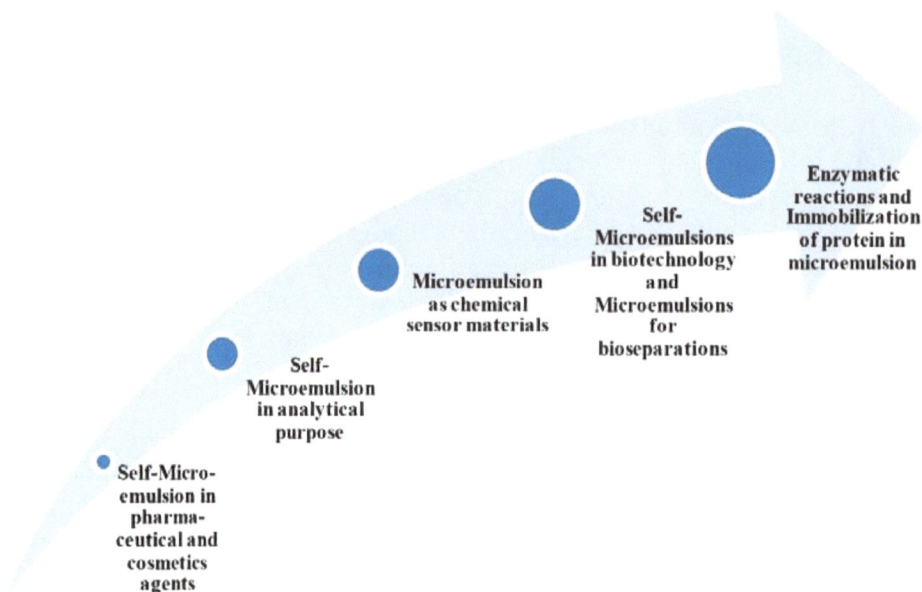

Fig. (2). Applications of SMEDDS in various fields.

Self-microemulsions in Pharmaceutical

Liquid crystalline, micellar and emulsion creating systems are generally utilized as a part of pharmaceutical products. The simple formulation, remarkable environment stability, admirable solubilization limit and so on favor MEs to be an excellent suggestion over other formulation systems. The dispersed phase, hydrophobic or hydrophilic can act as a potential reservoir for drugs that can be partitioned among dispersed and continuous phases. Interacting with a semipermeable layer, for example, skin or mucous film, the drug can be transferred *via* a barrier.

Less viscous preparations with appropriate protein compatible surfactants are injection solutions because they are miscible with blood in any proportion. While, emulsions and MEs result in less immunoreactions or fat embolism. Proteins are not denatured in MEs even though they are not stable at low or high temperatures. The aggregate dosage of the drug can be diminished when used as ME and hence reactions can be limited. Toxicity and bio-incompatibility of ingredients are important parameters for development of effective formulation.

A utilization of o/w ME in the pharmaceutical market is the use of lipophilic fluorocarbons (as oils) to make short time blood plasma substitutes to keep up the delivery of oxygen in living systems. The parts to be utilized must have short hypersensitive activity, extraordinary compatibility with physiology of the body and high biocompatibility. Lecithins and non-ionic surfactants fulfill the biocompatibility that is essential for amphiphiles.

Fortovase, Kaletra, Targretin, Vesanoid, Gengraf, Lipirex, Solufen are some examples of marketed products of SEDDS which show their utility in pharmaceutical.

Emulsion (o/w type) has been fabricated for oral intake of insulin using surfactant-coated insulin which demonstrated enhanced efficacy after oral administration. Poly(*iso*-butyl cyanoacrylate) nanocapsules dispersed in a biocompatible ME showed considerable lessening in glucose levels in diabetic rats than the solution of insulin [37].

Garcia-Celma 45 has reviewed MEs as DDS for various types of drugs such as anti-cancer (doxorubicin, idarubicin, tetrabenzamidine derivative), sympatholytics (bupranolol, timolol, levobunolol, propanolol), anti-infective (cloitrimazole, ciclopirox olamine, econazole nitrate, tetracycline HCl), peptide (cyclosporine, insulin, vassopressin), NSAIDS (butibufen, indomethacin), steroids (testosterone, testosterone propionate, testosterone enanthate, progesterone, medroxyprogestoraneacetate), local anesthetics (lidocaine, benzocaine, tetracaine, heptacaine), anxiolytics (benzodiazepines), vitamins (menadione, ascorbic acid) and dermological (tyrocine, azelaic acid) [38]. Enzyme doped silica nanoparticles in the aqueous portion of reverse micelles and diospyrin microencapsulated; bisnapthoquinol is a drug that has a possible chemotherapeutic response that has been established as formulation [39].

Cosmetics Agents as Self-microemulsions

It is assumed that microemulsion formulations will result in fast retention of drug into the skin. Costs, security, appropriate segment assurance are the main perspectives in the formulations of microemulsions. Healthy skin microemulsions comprise of surfactants, cosurfactants and oils such as sodium alkyl sulfate, dodecyl oligoglucoside, transcutol, lecithin, propanol, alkyl dimethyl amine oxide, hexadecane, isopropyl myristate and amino-utilitarian poly-organosiloxane and acid or furthermore a salt of the metal.

A cosmetic ME of silicone oil was developed by the emulsion polymerization technique. Ultrafine emulsions generated by condensation techniques have a couple of great benefits in cosmetic and therapeutic products as they have fabulous stability and security and their globule size can be expeditiously regulated. These are o/w emulsions with globule estimates like microemulsion due to which they can be seen as thermodynamically unstable. Tokuoka *et al.,* thought about the solubilization of different systems involving water, surfactant and synthetic scents (d-limonene, ionone, benzyl acetate, eugenol, hexylcinnamaldehyde and linalol), clarifying:

a. The effect of fragrance on the areas of ternary phase.
b. The distribution coefficient among the bulk phase and micelles.
c. The partition among dissolved and solubilized aroma relying on their volatility [40].

Oligoglucoside, propanol, IPM, hexadecane, lecithin, alkyldimethylaminesulfate and sodium alkyl sulphate are used for skin care products as ME formulations [41]. Fragrance and flavored oils are also incorporated in these formulations. Temperature and vapor pressure over time is investigated as a critical parameter for the cosmetic utilization of MEs [42].

These are also used in transdermal drug delivery such as the use of curcumin for the treatment of a variety of diseases such as skin cancer, psoriasis and scleroderma [43]. They can be considered as an appropriate carrier system for the functioning of ascorbic acid as a whitening agent. MEs containing transcutol established the best preparation to convey the entire dose and also improved permeability through the skin [44]. This demonstrated the best outcomes in having anti-fungal potential against *Candida albicans*. Hence, these types of MEs show potential for clinical investigation. Betamethasone dipropionate and salicylic acid loaded ME gels offered good anti-inflammatory potential for the ailment of psoriasis [45].

Analytical Purpose of Self-microemulsions

Microemulsions are used as a piece of the field of analytical methodologies such as chromatography, laser-excited photoionization spectroscopy, *etc.* In microemulsion electrokinetic chromatography (MEEKC), assessment of solute hydrophobicity was finished, which gives a speedy and reproducible methodology to procure hydrophobic factors for solvents. MEs can improve diagnostic spectroscopic procedures. MEs are used in three frameworks such as w/o, o/w and bicontinuous. MEs have been analyzed in analytical spectroscopy and analytical sensitivities. Both microemulsion and mixed microemulsion structures have been utilized for a sequence of analyses for the identification of copper, aluminum, cadmium, zinc and manganese particles. Chinese Chemical Society published these investigations in the Journals [46].

MEs (o/w) are utilized in reversed-phase chromatography because of the high amount of water and MEs (w/o) with a high amount of oil which is suitable for normal-phase chromatography. SLS is generally used as a surfactant and butan-1-

ol as a co-surfactant. Heptane and octane are the most commonly used oils.

Soil treatment has been reported using rapeseed methyl loaded MEs for extraction of a variety of components from soil such as polychlorinated biphenyls and polycyclic aromatic hydrocarbons by using chlorinated hydrocarbons and hydrophilic surfactants. Pesticides (o/w and w/o) are utilized for the elimination of impurities and detoxification of mustard compounds. These are also utilized for measuring the presence of polycyclic aromatic hydrocarbon by phosphorescence [47].

Self-microemulsions for Biotechnology

Starting late, excitement on MEs is being used for a variety of uses in biotechnology such as enzymatic actions, immobilization and bioseparation of proteins. These are superior to other multiphase equilibrium structures due to their instant solubilization of polar and non-polar reactants in the same media, moving of balanced position of reaction and partition of things by physical strategies. Regardless, the bio-incompatibility of used amphiphiles is bonafide in the progress of this area.

The prospects of biotechnological usage are being watched carefully. Protein reactions in ME media have been widely considered. Their utilization for protein catalysis isn't discretionary for enzyme under *in vivo* state in the cell and at the interface of lipophilic and lipophobic spaces of cell and tissue comprising of lipidic and other basic amphiphiles [48, 49].

Use of Microemulsions in Enzymatic Reactions

The potential good conditions of using enzymes in w/o MEs are:

i. Expanded solvency of non-polar reactants.
ii. Chances of altering thermodynamic equilibria for condensation.
iii. Thermal stability increment of enzyme, authorizing reaction to be conducted at a higher temperature.

Catalysis by an enormous amount of the enzymes in ME media has been inspected for a number of reactions such as the blend of esters, transesterifications, glycerolysis, distinctive hydrolysis reactions, oxidation, peptides and sugar acetals, diminishment and transformation of steroids. The configuration and response of enzymes rely upon water/surfactant and the protein is sensitive to the proportion of surrounding water.

There is a variety of lipase ME systems for synthetic and hydrolytic reactions that demonstrate their potential in the field of biotechnology [50]. These are microemulsion-based gels that act as media for bio-organic reactions using lipases as a catalyst. Production of chiral epoxides employing *mycobacterium* in w/o emulsions is one of the stereochemical benefits of the ME [51]. Gomez-Puyon has conducted a study on the behavior of enzymes in MEs [52].

Microemulsion for Immobilization of Protein

This medium has been established to be a superior rank in the field of protein immobilization. Immobilization of proteins on appropriate solid surfaces utilizing its media has been effectively done [53]. Candida rugosa lipase has been immobilized using gelatin-containing AOT microemulsion-based organogels and as well as silica gel [54].

Bioseparations by Microemulsions

The probabilities of MEs to separate biopolymers (catalysts) from the aqueous phase have been investigated. These are sensitive solvents for protein extraction without changing their enzymatic or utilitarian highlights, disregarding the ways this strategy can immediately be scaled by the traditional liquid-liquid extraction method. The pH, ionic quality, salt type, concentration of the solvent and temperature affect protein's partition [55 - 57].

Microemulsions as Chemical Sensor Materials

MEs as novel crystalline colloidal arrays (CCA) are novel innovations that are used as new chemical sensors by diffracting light scattering (Bragg's law) because these are mesoscopically discontinuous fluid compounds. A smart photoionic CCA self-assembly can be used for pharmaceutical, natural science, process control and remote recognizing. They assemble into either FCC or BCC frame. Essentially as nuclear atomic stones diffract X-beams that obey the Bragg law, CCAs diffract light.

Colloidal components of inorganic mixes, for example, silica or organic polymers like poly (N-isopropylacrylamide) have been explored having the range of approximately 200 nm. A propelled detecting material from a polymerized CCA was developed by Asher *et al.* This is a mesoscopically incidental CCA of circular polystyrene colloids inside a thin, smart polymer hydrogel film. Crown ether was used as the recognition remote to produce a sensor. This sensor can recognize the lead ions. The sensors for identification of glucose and galactose use glucose oxidase or fe-D-galactosidase as identifying elements. Other than detecting glucose, it can evaluate the concentration of oxygen in the existence of a glucose level.

Fabrication of thermally tunable photonic gem of PNIPAM, a novel CCA photoionic gem is produced that is used for molecular recognition procedures. For example, antibody/antigen interactions have been endeavored [58].

Microemulsions as Microreactors and Blood Substitutes

These are used as drug delivery vehicles due to their variety of potential and extraordinary advantages. They are used as an oral solid dosage form in micro-reactor and blood substitute form [59, 60].

DOSAGE FORM OF SMEDDS

Their marketed products are available in various dosage forms which include-

Oral Route

Oral route of LBDDS includes various dosage forms which are described below:

SE Capsules

After ingestion of capsules containing simple liquids in SE formulations, ME globules are formed and scattered in the GIT to achieve the site of assimilation. Irreversible partitioning of phase in ME results in the change of medicaments assimilation that can't be predictable. For taking care of this issue, sodium dodecyl sulfate is included in the SE formulation.

SE Sustained/Controlled Release

The blend of lipids, surfactant and polymer demonstrated an incredible potential for the formulation of SE controlled release formulations. These are of remarkable usefulness in forestalling antagonistic impact. The addition of indomethacin (or other NSAIDS) into this may enhance its efficiency *via* GI mucosal layer, conceivably lessening GI bleeding.

SE Pellets

Pellets have numerous points of interest over traditional solid dosage formulation such as manufacturing flexibility, decreasing inter/intrasubject variability of plasma profile and limiting irritation in GI without bringing down drug bioavailability.

SE Solid Dispersions

SDs could enhance the rate of dissolution and bioavailability of inadequately water-soluble drugs, butsome issues in their production and stability still exist. Serajuddin *et al.*, brought up that these troubles could be overcomed by the utilization of SE ingredients in SD [61].

Topical Delivery

These have a brilliant capability to transport a huge quantity of water and topical agents into the skin, higher than the capability of water alone or other conventional vehicles like lotions and creams, as they are an outstanding reservoir for PWS drugs for their capacity of improved solubilization such as miconazole nitrate loaded microemulsion [62]. Clotrimazole and fluconazole loaded microemulsion-based gels were formulated and compared with the commercially available gel of clotrimazole by *in vitro* methods [63]. They have received great significance in transdermal drug delivery. Topical delivery of drugs can have preferences over different techniques for a few reasons, among them one is escaping of the first-pass metabolism of medicaments and its associated toxicity impact.

Ocular Delivery

In traditional ophthalmic products, aqueous soluble drugs are fabricated in a solution. Aqueous insoluble drugs are fabricated as ointments or suspensions. Some major disadvantages of these systems are lack of effectiveness in posterior part of ocular tissue and low bioavailability in the corneal area. In recent research, significant efforts are being made by developing innovative and more efficient delivery systems. Microemulsion has come into spotlight as a possible dosage form for the ocular delivery of drugs.

Parental Delivery

Parental delivery of drugs with constrained solubility is a notable issue in industry in light of the low solubility of drugs conveyed on the target site [61].

Nasal Delivery

In recent times, the microemulsion has been investigated to improve the uptake of drugs across the nasal mucosa. Incorporation of a muco-adhesive polymer facilitates prolong transition time on mucosa. For administration of diazepam *via* the nasal route might be a beneficial technique for quick action in case of emergency ailment for epileptics.

Drug Targeting

Diseased cells can be targeted to know the existence of a variety of receptors, antigens/proteins which may be distinctively showed or overexpressed in these cells in contrast to the healthy cells. Specific antibodies and ligands can be utilized for targeting particular cells. Their less particle size provides an excellent chance to defeat the physiological obstacles and facilitate theefficient cellular absorption *via* intracellular internalization [64 - 66].

CONSENT FOR PUBLICATION

Not applicable.

CONFLICT OF INTEREST

The author declares no conflict of interest, financial or otherwise.

ACKNOWLEDGEMENTS

Declared none.

REFERENCES

[1]   Verma R, Kaushik D. *In vitro* lipolysis as a tool for establishment of IVIVC for lipid based drug delivery systems. Curr Drug Deliv 2019; 16(8): 688-97.
        [http://dx.doi.org/10.2174/1567201816666190620115716] [PMID: 31250755]

[2]   Dokania S, Joshi AK. Self-microemulsifying drug delivery system (SMEDDS)--challenges and road ahead. Drug Deliv 2015; 22(6): 675-90.
        [http://dx.doi.org/10.3109/10717544.2014.896058] [PMID: 24670091]

[3]   Eccleston GM. Emulsions and microemulsions. In: Swarbrick J, Ed. Encyclopedia of Pharm Techno Informa. New York: Healthcare 2007; 3: pp. 1548-65.

[4]   Sun C, Gui Y, Hu R, *et al.* Preparation and pharmacokinetics evaluation of solid self-microemulsifying drug delivery system (s-SMEDDS) of osthole. AAPS PharmSciTech 2018; 19(5): 2301-10.
        [http://dx.doi.org/10.1208/s12249-018-1067-3] [PMID: 29845504]

[5]   Agarwal V, Alayoubi A, Siddiqui A, Nazzal S. Powdered self-emulsified lipid formulations of meloxicam as solid dosage forms for oral administration. Drug Dev Ind Pharm 2012; 3(4): 1-9.
        [PMID: 23072611]

[6]   Yetukuri K, Sudheer P. Approaches to development of solid-self micron emulsifying drug delivery system: Formulation techniques and dosage forms: A review. Int J Pharm Sci Res 2012; 3(10): 3550-63.

[7]   Cerpnjak K, Zvonar A, Gašperlin M, Vrečer F. Lipid-based systems as a promising approach for enhancing the bioavailability of poorly water-soluble drugs. Acta Pharm 2013; 63(4): 427-45.
        [http://dx.doi.org/10.2478/acph-2013-0040] [PMID: 24451070]

[8]   Ke WT, Lin SY, Ho HO, Sheu MT. Physical characterizations of microemulsion systems using tocopheryl polyethylene glycol 1000 succinate (TPGS) as a surfactant for the oral delivery of protein drugs. J Control Release 2005; 102(2): 489-507.
        [http://dx.doi.org/10.1016/j.jconrel.2004.10.030] [PMID: 15653166]

[9]   Nornoo AO, Zheng H, Lopes LB, Johnson-Restrepo B, Kannan K, Reed R. Oral microemulsions of paclitaxel: *in situ* and pharmacokinetic studies. Eur J Pharm Biopharm 2009; 71(2): 310-7.
[http://dx.doi.org/10.1016/j.ejpb.2008.08.015] [PMID: 18793723]

[10]   Kim HJ, Yoon KA, Hahn M, Park ES, Chi SC. Preparation and *in vitro* evaluation of self-microemulsifying drug delivery systems containing idebenone. Drug Dev Ind Pharm 2000; 26(5): 523-9.
[http://dx.doi.org/10.1081/DDC-100101263] [PMID: 10789064]

[11]   Jadhav KR, Shaikh IM, Ambade KW, Kadam VJ. Applications of microemulsion based drug delivery system. Curr Drug Deliv 2006; 3(3): 267-73.
[http://dx.doi.org/10.2174/156720106777731118] [PMID: 16848728]

[12]   Kumar A, Sharma S, Kamble R. Self-emulsifying drug delivery system (SEDDS): Future aspects. Int J Pharm Pharm Sci 2010; 2(4): 7-13.

[13]   Verma A, Singh MK, Kumar B. Development and characterization of Flutamide containing self micro emulsifying drug delivery system (SMEDDS). Int J Pharm Pharm Sci 2011; 3(4): 60-5.

[14]   Dahan A, Hoffman A. Rationalizing the selection of oral lipid based drug delivery systems by an *in vitro* dynamic lipolysis model for improved oral bioavailability of poorly water soluble drugs. J Control Release 2008; 129(1): 1-10.
[http://dx.doi.org/10.1016/j.jconrel.2008.03.021] [PMID: 18499294]

[15]   Chakraborty S, Shukla D, Mishra B, Singh S. Lipid--an emerging platform for oral delivery of drugs with poor bioavailability. Eur J Pharm Biopharm 2009; 73(1): 1-15.
[http://dx.doi.org/10.1016/j.ejpb.2009.06.001] [PMID: 19505572]

[16]   Gursoy RN, Benita S. Self-emulsifying drug delivery systems (SEDDS) for improved oral delivery of lipophilic drugs. Biomed Pharmacother 2004; 58(3): 173-82.
[http://dx.doi.org/10.1016/j.biopha.2004.02.001] [PMID: 15082340]

[17]   Pouton CW, Charman WN. The potential of oily formulations for drug delivery to the gastrointestinal tract: preface. Adv Drug Deliv Rev 1997; 25(1): 1-2.
[http://dx.doi.org/10.1016/S0169-409X(96)00486-3] [PMID: 11733114]

[18]   Humberstone AJ, Charman WN. Lipid-based vehicles for the oral delivery of poorly water-soluble drugs. Adv Drug Deliv Rev 1997; 25(1): 103-28.
[http://dx.doi.org/10.1016/S0169-409X(96)00494-2]

[19]   Di Maio S, Carrier RL. Gastrointestinal contents in fasted state and post-lipid ingestion: *in vivo* measurements and *in vitro* models for studying oral drug delivery. J Control Release 2011; 151(2): 110-22.
[http://dx.doi.org/10.1016/j.jconrel.2010.11.034] [PMID: 21134406]

[20]   Cui SX, Nie SF, Li L, Wang CG, Pan WS, Sun JP. Preparation and evaluation of self-microemulsifying drug delivery system containing vinpocetine. Drug Dev Ind Pharm 2009; 35(5): 603-11.
[http://dx.doi.org/10.1080/03639040802488089] [PMID: 19040178]

[21]   Verma R, Mittal V, Kaushik D. Self-microemulsifying drug delivery system: A vital approach for bioavailability enhancement. Int J Chemtech Res 2017; 10(7): 515-28.

[22]   Kumar A, Nanda A. Design and optimization of ezetimibe self microemulsifying drug delivery system for enhanced therapeutic potential. Drug Deliv Lett 2018; 8(3): 248-57.
[http://dx.doi.org/10.2174/2210303108666180528074708]

[23]   Singh AK, Chaurasiya A, Singh M, Upadhyay SC, Mukherjee R, Khar RK. Exemestane loaded self-microemulsifying drug delivery system (SMEDDS): development and optimization. AAPS PharmSciTech 2008; 9(2): 628-34.
[http://dx.doi.org/10.1208/s12249-008-9080-6] [PMID: 18473177]

[24]   Akula S, Gurram AK, Devireddy SR. Self-microemulsifying drug delivery systems: An attractive strategy for enhanced therapeutic profile. Int Sch Res Notices 2014. Article ID 964051, 1-11

[25]   Ghosh PK, Majithiya RJ, Umrethia ML, Murthy RSR. Design and development of microemulsion drug delivery system of acyclovir for improvement of oral bioavailability. AAPS PharmSciTech 2006; 7(3): 77.
[http://dx.doi.org/10.1208/pt070377] [PMID: 17025257]

[26]   Podlogar F, Gasperlin M, Tomsic M, Jamnik A, Rogac MB. Structural characterisation of water-Tween 40/Imwitor 308-isopropyl myristate microemulsions using different experimental methods. Int J Pharm 2004; 276(1-2): 115-28.
[http://dx.doi.org/10.1016/j.ijpharm.2004.02.018] [PMID: 15113620]

[27]   Khadka P, Ro J, Kim H, *et al.* Pharmaceutical particle technologies: An approach to improve drug solubility, dissolution and bioavailability. Asian J Pharm Sci 2014; 9(6): 304-16.
[http://dx.doi.org/10.1016/j.ajps.2014.05.005]

[28]   Bagwe RP, Kanicky JR, Palla BJ, Patanjali PK, Shah DO. Improved drug delivery using microemulsions: rationale, recent progress, and new horizons. Crit Rev Ther Drug Carrier Syst 2001; 18(1): 77-140.
[PMID: 11326744]

[29]   Parmar N, Singla N, Amin S, Kohli K. Study of cosurfactant effect on nanoemulsifying area and development of lercanidipine loaded (SNEDDS) self nanoemulsifying drug delivery system. Colloids Surf B Biointerfaces 2011; 86(2): 327-38.
[http://dx.doi.org/10.1016/j.colsurfb.2011.04.016] [PMID: 21550214]

[30]   Rahman MA, Hussain A, Hussain MS, Mirza MA, Iqbal Z. Role of excipients in successful development of self-emulsifying/microemulsifying drug delivery system (SEDDS/SMEDDS). Drug Dev Ind Pharm 2013; 39(1): 1-19.
[http://dx.doi.org/10.3109/03639045.2012.660949] [PMID: 22372916]

[31]   Verma R, Kaushik D. Design and optimization of candesartan loaded self-nanoemulsifying drug delivery system for improving its dissolution rate and pharmacodynamic potential 2020.
[http://dx.doi.org/10.1080/10717544.2020.1760961]

[32]   Anton N, Vandamme TF. Nano-emulsions and micro-emulsions: clarifications of the critical differences. Pharm Res 2011; 28(5): 978-85.
[http://dx.doi.org/10.1007/s11095-010-0309-1] [PMID: 21057856]

[33]   Rao J, McClements DJ. Food-grade microemulsions and nanoemulsions: Role of oil phase composition on formation and stability. Food Hydrocoll 2012; 29: 326-34.
[http://dx.doi.org/10.1016/j.foodhyd.2012.04.008]

[34]   Agrawal S, Giri TK, Tripathi DK, Alexander A. A review on novel therapeutic strategies for the enhancement of solubility for hydrophobic drugs through lipid and surfactant based self micro emulsifying drug delivery system: A novel approach. Am J Drug Disc Dev 2012; 2(4): 143-83.
[http://dx.doi.org/10.3923/ajdd.2012.143.183]

[35]   Gahlawat N, Verma R, Kaushik D. Recent Developments in self-microemulsifying drug delivery system: An overview. Asian J Pharm 2019; 13(2): 59-72.

[36]   Bharti D, Pandey P, Verma R, Kaushik D. Development and characterization of rosuvastatin loaded self-emulsifying drug delivery system. Appl Clin Res Clin Trials Regul Aff 2018; 5: 1-8.
[http://dx.doi.org/10.2174/2213476X05666180309160113]

[37]   Patil NH, Devarajan PV. Colloidal carriers for noninvasive delivery of insulin. Colloid and Interface Science in Pharmaceutical Research and Development 2014; 4: 600-23.
[http://dx.doi.org/10.1016/B978-0-444-62614-1.00020-X]

[38]   Solans C, Kunieda H, Eds. Industrial applications of microemulsions, Marcel Dekker Inc., New York, 1997; Tadros Th F, p. 199; Dungan SR, pp. 147–174; Gasco, MR, pp. 97–122; Garcia-Celma, MJ, pp.

123–145; Holmberg K, pp. 69–95

[39] Jain TK, Roy I, De TK, Maitra AN. J Am Chem Soc 1998; 120: 11092-2.
      [http://dx.doi.org/10.1021/ja973849x]

[40] Tokuokas Y, Uchiyama H, Abe M, Christian SD. Langmuir 1995; 11: 725.
      [http://dx.doi.org/10.1021/la00003a010]

[41] Rhee YS, Park CW, Nam TY, Shin YS, Chi SC, Park ES. Formulation of parenteral microemulsion
      containing itraconazole. Arch Pharm Res 2007; 30(1): 114-23.
      [http://dx.doi.org/10.1007/BF02977787] [PMID: 17328251]

[42] Sharma A, Garg T, Aman A, *et al.* Nanogel-an advanced drug delivery tool: Current and future. Artif
      Cells Nanomed Biotechnol 2014; 1: 1-13.

[43] Joshi D, Garg T, Goyal AK, Rath G. Advanced drug delivery approaches against periodontitis. Drug
      Deliv 2014; 1-15.
      [PMID: 25005586]

[44] Joshi D, Garg T, Goyal AK, Rath G. Development and characterization of novel medicated nanofibers
      against Periodontitis. Curr Drug Deliv 2014; 4(1): 56-72.
      [PMID: 25488417]

[45] Kalia V, Garg T, Rath G, Goyal AK. Development and evaluation of a sublingual film of the
      antiemetic granisetron hydrochloride. Artif Cells Nanomed Biotechnol 2014; 1-5.
      [http://dx.doi.org/10.3109/21691401.2014.984303] [PMID: 25435408]

[46] Guo R, Zhu XJ. Chin Univer 1987; 8: 508-15.

[47] Sharma R, Singh H, Joshi M, *et al.* Recent advances in polymeric electrospun nanofibers for drug
      delivery. Crit Rev Ther Drug Carrier Syst 2014; 31(3): 187-217.
      [http://dx.doi.org/10.1615/CritRevTherDrugCarrierSyst.2014008193] [PMID: 24940748]

[48] Kaur V, Garg T, Rath G, Goyal AK. Therapeutic potential of nanocarrier for overcoming to P-
      glycoprotein. J Drug Target 2014; 22(10): 859-70.
      [http://dx.doi.org/10.3109/1061186X.2014.947295] [PMID: 25101945]

[49] Malik R, Garg T, Goyal AK, Rath G. Polymeric nanofibers: targeted gastro-retentive drug delivery
      systems. J Drug Target 2014; 4(8): 1-16.
      [PMID: 25268275]

[50] Modgill V, Garg T, Goyal AK, Rath G. Permeability study of ciprofloxacin from ultra-thin
      nanofibrous film through various mucosal membranes. Artif Cells Nanomed Biotechnol 2014; 1-6.
      [PMID: 24915047]

[51] Morie A, Garg T, Goyal AK, Rath G. Nanofibers as novel drug carrier- an overview. Artif Cells
      Nanomed Biotechnol 2014; 1-9.
      [PMID: 25016918]

[52] Gomez-Puyon A, Ed. Biomol. Org. Solvents, CRC Press, Boca Raton, 1992; 7:540-60

[53] Holmberg K, Bergstrom K, Brink C, *et al.* Adhesion Sci Technol 1993; 7: 503-25.
      [http://dx.doi.org/10.1163/156856193X00826]

[54] Pabreja S, Garg T, Rath G, Goyal AK. Mucosal vaccination against tuberculosis using Ag85A-loaded
      immunostimulating complexes. Artif Cells Nanomed Biotechnol 2014; 5: 1-8.
      [PMID: 25307269]

[55] Reddy PUM, Babu PR, Rao PM, Edukondalu V, Mallikharjunarao KLN. Int J Res Pharm Nano Sci
      2013; 2(3): 317-31.

[56] Kelley BD, Wang DIC, Hatton TA. Affinity-based reversed micellar protein extraction: I. principles
      and protein-ligand systems. Biotechnol Bioeng 1993; 42(10): 1199-208.
      [http://dx.doi.org/10.1002/bit.260421010] [PMID: 18609669]

[57]   Adachi M, Harada M, Shioi A, Sato Y. J Phys Chem 1991; 95: 7925-52.
        [http://dx.doi.org/10.1021/j100173a068]

[58]   Asher SA, Kimble KW, Walker JP. Enabling thermoreversible physically cross-linked polymerized
        colloidal array photonic crystals. Chem Mater 2008; 20(24): 7501-9.
        [http://dx.doi.org/10.1021/cm801519x] [PMID: 19966904]

[59]   Sharma R, Garg T, Goyal AK, Rath G. Development, optimization and evaluation of polymeric
        electrospun nanofiber: A tool for local delivery of fluconazole for management of vaginal candidiasis.
        Artif Cells Nanomed Biotechnol 2014; 1: 1-8.
        [PMID: 25315503]

[60]   Shi FF, Bulkowski M, Hsieh KC. Synthesis of indium nanoclusters and formation of thin film contacts
        on plastic substrates for organic and flexible electronics applications. Nanotechnology 2007; 18(26):
        265301-12.
        [http://dx.doi.org/10.1088/0957-4484/18/26/265301] [PMID: 21730395]

[61]   Serajuddin AT. Solid dispersion of poorly water-soluble drugs: early promises, subsequent problems,
        and recent breakthroughs. J Pharm Sci 1999; 88(10): 1058-66.
        [http://dx.doi.org/10.1021/js980403l] [PMID: 10514356]

[62]   Hussain T, Garg T, Goyal AK, Rath G. Biomedical applications of nanofiber scaffolds in tissue
        engineering. J Biomater Tissue Eng 2014; 4(34): 23-32.
        [http://dx.doi.org/10.1166/jbt.2014.1214]

[63]   Johal HS, Garg T, Rath G, Goyal AK. Advanced topical drug delivery system for the management of
        vaginal candidiasis. Drug Deliv 2014; 1(2): 1-14.
        [PMID: 24959937]

[64]   Nigade PM, Patil SL, Tiwari SS. Self-emulsifying drug delivery system (SEDDS): A review. Int J
        Pharma Bio Sci 2012; 2(2): 42-52.

[65]   Pattewar SKS, Pande V, Sharma S. Self microemulsifying drug delivery system: A lipid-based drug
        delivery system. Int J Pharm Sci Res 2016; 7(2): 443-52.

[66]   Maulik J, Patel SSP, Natvarlal M, Patel MM. A Self-microemulsifying drug delivery system
        (SMEDDS). Int J Pharm Sci Rev Res 2010; 4(3): 29-35.

[67]   Gupta S, Kesarla R, Omri A. Formulation strategies to improve the bioavailability of poorly absorbed
        drugs with special emphasis on self-emulsifying systems. ISRN Pharm 2013; 2013(4)848043
        [http://dx.doi.org/10.1155/2013/848043] [PMID: 24459591]

CHAPTER 4

Components of Self-Microemulsifying Drug Delivery System

Ravinder Verma[1], Deepak Kaushik[1,*], Manish Kumar[2] and Deepak Parmar[3]

[1] Department of Pharmaceutical Sciences, Maharshi Dayanand University, Rohtak (Haryana), 124001, India

[2] M.M. College of Pharmacy, Mullana, Ambala, Haryana, India

[3] Department of Chemistry, Maharshi Dayanand University, Rohtak (Haryana), 124001, India

Abstract: The key thought in choosing suitable ingredients for any lipid-based formulations (LBFs) is the identification of an ingredient or their combination that can keep the whole drug dose in solubilized form for oral administration. The chief ingredients in LBFs are lipids, surfactant and co-surfactant that are described in detail. These components are meant for achieving the maximum drug loading, minimal time for self-emulsification and small size of globule in the gastric environment for obtaining maximum assimilation, lessening variation in the emulsion globule size and preventing or minimizing drug degradation. Generally, a low dose of the drug is appropriate for SMEDDS. Lipids are an important component in SMEDDS because they are responsible for fluidization of intestinal cell membrane, solubilization of hydrophobic drugs, enhancing the dissolution rate and solubility in GI fluids, protection of the drug from chemical and enzymatic degradation. Surfactants play an important role in enhancing the solubility of a hydrophobic drug in oil, dispersion of liquid vehicle in GIT fluids, improving bioavailability by increasing permeability, avoiding the precipitation of drug in GI lumen and prolonging the existence of drug moiety in a solubilized form that results in its effective assimilation. But, a few surfactants are orally acceptable. The combination of ionic and non-ionic surfactants is very effective for improving the degree/area of the micro-emulsion region. It plays an important role in the synergetic effect in critical micelle concentration. A high amount of surfactant is essential to diminish interfacial tension adequately, which can cause gastric irritation, otherwise. That is why; co-surfactants of HLB value 10-14 are added to reduce their concentration. They are added in combination with surfactants to provide sufficient flexibility to interfacial film, dissolve a greater quantity of either hydrophobic drug or hydrophilic surfactant in the lipidic base and decreasing the interface of oil/water. They help in dissolving a large amount of surfactant or drug in lipid base, assisting the dispersion process, decreasing the amount of surfactant in the formulation and perform-

---

* **Corresponding author Deepak Kaushik:** Department of Pharmaceutical Sciences, Maharshi Dayanand University, Rohtak (Haryana), 124001, India; Tel: +91 9315809626; E-mail: deepkaushik1977@gmail.com

ing an action of co-surfactant in microemulsion system. This chapter highlights the various categories of ingredients that are used in the formulation of SMEDDS and their marketed products.

Keywords: Co-surfactant, HLB value, Lipids, Multi-functional excipients, Surfactants, SMEDDS.

SELECTION OF INGREDIENTS IN SEFS

The key thought in choosing suitable ingredients for any LBFs is the identification of an ingredient or their combination that can keep the complete drug dose in the solubilized form in a volume adequate for oral administration. The self-emulsification process depends upon the type of the oil/surfactant combination, the concentration of surfactant, oil/surfactant ratio, and the temperature at which self-emulsification exists. In favor of these statements, it has also been shown that very specific mixtures of the ingredients could result in efficient self-emulsifying systems (SEFs). The drug must be chemically and physically stable in the preparation and drug discharge features should be stable during the shelf-life of the product. Another requirement is the physical and chemical stability of ingredients that should be cautiously observed during the development of formulation. The ingredient should be selected from the catalog of "Generally Regarded as Safe" (GRAS) ingredients [1]. The chief ingredients in SESs are lipids, surfactant and co-surfactant, as shown in Fig. (**1**).

The combination of Pharmaceutical ingredients leads to proficient self-emulsifying formulations. These components are meant for achieving maximum drug loading, minimal time for self emulsification and globule size in gastric milieu for obtaining maximum assimilation, lessening variation in globule size and preventing or minimizing the drug degradation. For the selection of an appropriate SE vehicle, the following are to be addressed:

a. The drug solubility in a variety of ingredients.
b. Self-emulsifying region in the phase diagram.
c. Particle size distribution after the SE process.

Solubility is a useful parameter for the choice of a solvent for a specific purpose. The solubility factor suggests the compatibility between the two ingredients. Hildebrand solubility parameters are useful for the prediction of the formulation features.

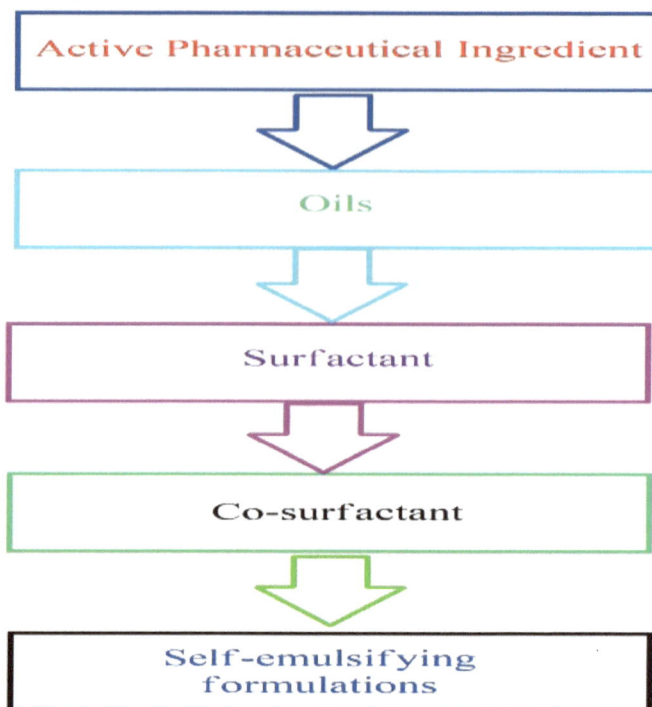

Fig. (1). Various components/ingredients of the self-emulsifying system.

Hydrophilic-Lipophilic Balance (HLB)

An empirical rule of HLB is utilized for the characterization of surfactants and the selection of suitable surfactants for the development of microemulsions in for a particular drug.

Partition Coefficient

The hydrophobicity of a compound is related to the partition coefficient of a molecule. Hydrophobic and lipophobic phase is also an important factor in the selection of ingredients. Molecules with the log P value greater than 4 are more soluble in oils and the molecules with the intermediate log P value (less than 4) may need a combination of hydrophilic surfactants (HLB 4-12) to create an SES with the highest solubility. Molecules with a low log P value shows the highest solubility in oil phase, while a compound with high log P value does not show the highest solubility in oil [2].

IDENTIFICATION OF SUITABLE DRUG CANDIDATE FOR SEDDS

Generally, a low dose of the drug is appropriate for SMEDDS. The solubility of the drug and polarity of lipidic phase are essential parameters. The polarity relies on HLB value, chain length and unsaturation of FAs. Maintenance of drug solubility in the GIT is the primary task for any oral preparation and maximizing drug solubility at the site of assimilation in the gut. For hydrophobic drug molecules that show limited dissolution-rate assimilation, SEDDS are the best choice, as they improve the rate and extent of assimilation, resulting in reproducible blood time profiles [3].

The drug is the most important ingredient for formulations. The drug must be soluble in the lipidic phase, as this feature of drug is important for maintaining the drug in the solubilized state. Drugs having a very high dose and low solubility in oil are not suitable for SMEDDS formulation. Drugs having a greater melting point with a log P value of 2 are rarely appropriate for these formulations. Hydrophobic drugs with log P value of more than 5 are suitable drugs for these formulations [4].

Utilization of SESs can be exploited to all four classes of BCS class drugs. They can help out in resolving the troubles of all these drugs. Rule of five was given by Lipinski that has been broadly used as a qualitative predictive model for oral assimilation profile. In innovation, the "rule of five indicates poor assimilation or poor permeability when there are more than five H-bond donors and H-bond acceptors, the molecular weight is < 500 Daltons and the log P value is < 5."

Although this rule is helpful at the initial screening phase but it has its limitations too. It should be considered that it is only applicable for compounds that are not substrates for active transporters and with the growing number of facts signifying that most drugs are substrates for a number of efflux or uptake transporters, this restriction might be distinguished. Log P value alone is improbably adequate for recognizing the appropriateness of LBFs because they do not effectively guess *in vivo* potential. It has been established that PWS candidates are commonly categorized as hydrophobic, they act in different ways in similar vehicles, thus highlighting the requirement of evaluating ingredients on an individual basis [5].

COMPONENTS OF SMEDDS

SMEDDS are composed of oil, surfactant and co-surfactant. The ratio of oil and surfactant concentration depends upon the solubility of the drug and self-emulsifying ability. The nature of oil, the concentration of surfactant and the temperature at which self emulsification occurs, are important factors during the formulation of SMEDDS [3].

Lipids/Oils

Lipids are also called oils, which assume an imperative part in SMEDDS because they are responsible for the solubilization of hydrophobic drug. For the most part, drugs utilized as a part of SMEDDS are hydrophilic in nature and have more noteworthy solubility in TGs than surfactants. The emulsification feature of oils relies on the molecular structure of the oil.

Selection of Oil

Strickley's survey discovered that in oral formulations, dietary oils of MCT (coconut, palm seed oil) or LCT such as corn, olive, nut, rapeseed, sesame, soyabean and hydrogenated vegetable oils are generally utilized as a part of SMEDDS because of their superior biocompatibility. Oils are utilized as a part of SMEDDS in the concentration range of around 40-80%. Modified and hydrolyzed vegetables are favored on the grounds that they demonstrate greater potential of solubility, and form a great self-emulsification system with a substantial number of surfactants supportive for an oral ingestion. They offer physiological and formulation stability and their debased items look like the final result of intestinal digestion. LCT is immiscible with hydrophilic surfactant and co-solvent. Mixed glycerides (polar oils) indicate an affinity towards hydrophilic surfactant and co-solvent, and help in the arrangement of self-dispersion formulation (SDF). Some examples of lipids commonly used as ingredients in SMEDDS are shown in Table **1**.

Table 1. Some examples of oils commonly employed as ingredients in SMEDDS.

S. No.	Commercial Name	Chemical Name	Regulatory Status
1.	Vegetable oil	Long-chain TAG	Oral product, GRAS, FDA IIG
2.	Capmul	Medium-chain TAG, caprylic/capric TAG	Oral product, GRAS, FDA IIG
3.	Captex 355	Glyceryl caprylate caprate	GRAS, FDA IIG
4.	Ethyl oleate	Ethyl ester of C18:1 omega FA	FDA IIG
5.	Maiscine 35-1	Glyceryl mono-linoleate	Oral product, GRAS, E471, EP, USP-NF
6.	Trcaprylin	Medium-chain TAG	-
7.	Labrafac CC	Caprylic/capric TG	-
8.	Isopropyl myristate	FA ester	FDA IIG
9.	Labrafac PG	PG dicaprylocaprate	USFA, JSFA, EP
10.	Peceol	Glyceryl mono-oleate	GRAS, E471, EP, USP-NF, FDA IIG
11.	Imwitor 988	Caprylic/capric glycerides	USP, Ph.Eur

(Table 1) cont.....

S. No.	Commercial Name	Chemical Name	Regulatory Status
12.	Akoline MCM	Caprylic/capric glycerides	-

Role

1. Use for fluidization of intestinal cell layer and opening of tight junction, which help in enhancing membrane permeability.

2. Enhance assimilation of drug by adding lipids in the formulation.

3. Expanding the rate of dissolution and solubility in GI liquids, and maintaining the security of drug from chemical and enzymatic degradation by changing in pharmaceutical features of drug.

4. Used to break lipophilic drugs, encourage self-emulsification and improve the amount of lipophilic drug transported *via* the lymphatic system by associating with core of the lipoprotein.

5. Along these lines, MCT or MCT with various degrees of saturation ought to be utilized to prepare SMEDDS [6, 7].

Lipids in Oral Drug delivery

Lipids alter their configuration and physiochemical features, digestibility and as well as the retention path. Accordingly, the determination of lipid ingredients and dosage form pronouncedly affect the drug assimilation and distribution [8]. Specifically, the associated features and performances of lipids can assume major parts:

Lipids possibly will have amphiphilic arrangements that decide their capacity of self-assembling in the fluid milieu. Such performance can critically affect drug disposition kinetics in GIT [9].

They can also act as solvents, prompting drug being available in GI fluids in this manner and avoiding the drug dissolution step.

When dietary and lipidic formulations are ingested, lipids digestion occurs that prompt the creation of colloidal micelles in the GIT, giving transient solubilization of drug and lessening chances for precipitation of drugs that affect its assimilation [10].

Methods of Controlled Discharge with Lipids

The controlled discharge systems can be abridged as matrix controlled discharge, gastro retention and stimulation of lymphatic transportation.

Matrix performs as an obstruction to a moderate manifestation of dissolved drug in GI fluids, by hindering diffusion or dissolution of the matrix prior to exposure of undissolved drug contents.

Gastroretention methods are used to maintain the drug in the solubilized form in the gastric milieu, anticipating transit before the total drug discharge. Prolonged assimilation coupled with moderate drug discharge can delay drug assimilation and its therapeutic impact. Drug transport through lymph is enhanced with expanding quantities of co-administered lipids. Lipids bind to the chylomicrons, that provide a prominent pool for the drugs in directly entering into the blood circulation. Such lymphatic transportation evades hepatic first-pass metabolism [11]. Solid lipid particles are made up of melt-emulsified lipids that are solid in nature. They prevent the organic solvents, resulting in a stable system having defensive effects against severe drug toxicity [9].

Slow degradation of the lipid manages *in vitro* discharge of drug by extending plasma residence and restrains peak plasma concentrations in contrast to other preparations [12].

Surfactants

Many chemicals that have surfactant-like features might be utilized for the formulation of SE systems; however, the choice is limited as too many surfactants are not orally acceptable. A surfactant is an amphiphilic agent that contains two sections. One section has a proclivity for water (polar solvents) and another part has proclivity for oil, broadly utilized as an emulsifying or solubilizing agent. These are being used to make more stable micro-emulsion. A mixture of ionic and non-ionic surfactants can be useful to increase the level of micro-emulsion area. They play a vital role in the development of colloidal sized cluster in the solution. They assemble at the interface of oil-water and settle at the internal stage (internal phase) in an emulsion. Anionic and non-ionic surfactant blend is responsible for synergetic impact in critical micelle concentration (CMC). Around 30-60% w/w of formulation of surfactants are utilized to create stable SMEDDS. There is a correlation between conc. of surfactant and droplet size, by expanding surfactant conc., the droplet estimate diminishes. Sometimes, the mean droplet size may increase by expanding conc. of surfactant. High quantities of surfactants can result in irritation in the GI tract. Surfactants acquired from natural origins are safer than synthetic or suggested for self-dispersed lipid formulation (SDLF), but they have a limited self-emulsification capability [13].

Non-ionic surfactants are recognized to be less harmful than ionic surfactants because they may cause direct reversible alterations in the intestinal wall. The high value of HLB and consequent hydrophilicity of surfactants is fundamental for the development of o/w globules as well as quick dispersion in the aqueous milieu, giving a decent scattering/SE activity. They are ready to be dissolved and solubilized at a moderate concentration to high amounts of the hydrophobic drug because of their amphiphilic nature. The prevention of precipitation inside the GI wall and the extended occurrence of the drug candidates in the solubilized state is very important for efficient retention. The lipid blends with higher surfactant and co-surfactant/oil proportions and prompts the development of SMEDDS [14 - 17]. There are various surfactants which are enlisted in Table **2**.

Table 2. Some examples of surfactants and co-surfactants commonly used as ingredients in SMEDDS.

S. No.	Marketed Name	Chemically	HLB	Regulatory Status
1.	Tween 85	Polyethylene (20) sorbitan trioleate	11	UK
2.	Labrafil M1944CS	Oleoyl macrogolglycerides	4	EP, FDA IIG, USP NF
3.	Labrafil M2125CS	Linoleoyl macrogolglycerides	4	EP, FDA IIG, USP NF
4.	Lauroglycol 90	PG monolaurate	5	USFA, FCC, EFA, USP-NF
5.	Vitamin Polysorbate 20/ Tween 20E TPGS	D-alpha-tocopheryl PEG 1000 succinate	13	Oral product
6.	Cremophor EL	Polyoxyl 35 castor oil	12-14	Oral product, USP-NF, FDA IIG
7.	Cremophor RH 40	Polyoxyl 40 hydrogenated castor oil	12-14	Oral product, USP-NF, FDA IIG
8.	Gelucire 44/14	Lauroyl macrogolglycerides	14	EP, USP-NF, FDA IIG
9.	Labrasol	Capylocaproyl macrogol glycerides	14	EP, USP-NF, FDA IIG
10.	Polysorbate 80	Polyoxyethylene sorbitan monooleate	15	Oral product, GRAS, EP, USP-NF, FDA IIG
11.	Tween 20	Polyoxyethylene sorbitan monolaurate	16.7	Oral product, GRAS, EP, USP-NF, FDA IIG

Mechanism

Interference of lipid bilayer of an epithelial membrane with unstirred watery layer forms the rate-limiting barrier to drug retention/diffusion and consequently inhibits the cytochrome P450. Lipophilicity of the surfactant demonstrates the effect on the emulsion that is formed after the assimilation of lipid. Surfactants with HLB >10 form finer and uniform globules in the microemulsion when contrasted with lipophilic surfactants with low HLB values. Most of the times, both the mixes of low and high HLB surfactants prompt development of stable microemulsion. Generally, the surfactants used for SEFs are water-soluble in nature. These are ester amphiphilic ingredients with medium to high HLB contingent on type and degree of esterification. Solid dosage type of LBFs may enhance the stability, yet having low drug loading and enormous potential for drug crystallization. Ethoxylated lipid surfactants such as Gelucire®, Labrasol® and Cremophor® had demonstrated that they retard the P-gp adjusted drug efflux [2].

Classification

Surfactants are categorized into four categories based on the hydrophilic group present in the molecules, which are:

Anionic Surfactants

These have a negative charge on a hydrophilic group such as carboxyl, sulphonate, sulphate, alkyl phenols and olefin sulphates. Example: Potassium laurate, sodium lauryl sulphate.

Cationic Surfactants

These have a positive charge on hydrophilic groups such as amines with amide linkages, polyethylene alkyl and alicyclic amines, polyoxyethylene fatty acid amides. Example: Quaternary ammonium halide.

Ampholytic Surfactants

These have both positive and negative charges on the hydrophilic group. Example: Sulfobetaines.

Non-ionic Surfactants

These have no charge on the hydrophilic group, but their derivatives have aqueous solubility from with highly polar groups like hydroxyl or polyethylene, polyoxyethylene glycol ester, polyoxyethylene fatty acid amides, carboxylic amides. Example: Spans, Tweens.

Classification Based on Hydrophilic-Lipophilic Balance (HLB) Number-

Lipophilic Surfactants

These have HLB value less than ten and have greater lipophilicity.

Hydrophilic Surfactants

These have HLB value greater than ten and have greater hydrophilicity.

Classification Based on the Composition of Counter-ion-

Monoatomic/Inorganic

(a) Cationic metal: Alkaline earth metal, alkali metal, transition metal

(b) Anions: Halides of bromide, chloride, iodide

Polyatomic/Organic

(a) Cations: Triethanolamine, ammonium, pyridinium,

(b) Anions: Tosyls, methyl sulphate [15].

Role

1. Upgrade solubilization of hydrophobic drug in oils.

2. Used to scatter liquid vehicle on dilution in GIT fluids. Consequently, oil/surfactant blend containing the drug is a type of fine globules which spread rapidly in GI tract

3. Enhance bioavailability by expanding permeability as they interfere with the lipidic bilayer of the epithelial cell membrane, which is deemed as a rate-constraining obstruction to drug retention/diffusion. Other mechanisms are upgrading rate of dissolution, improving tight junction's permeability or diminishing/repressing p-glycoprotein drug efflux

4. Upgrade the rate of dissolution of the formulation

5. Preventing precipitation inside the GI lumen and delayed presence of drug moiety in a soluble state, which is exceptionally capable of effective retention

6. The surface zone of the drug can be expanded by utilizing surfactants [16, 17].

Surfactants are chiefly utilized to enhance oral bioavailability. In case of ricinoleic acid, the existence of hydroxyl aggregate on the C-12 of ricinoleic acid, and glycerides consisting of unsaturated fat (Cremophor® EL) show ethoxylation and enhance the hydrophilicity and bioavailability. Surfactants can enhance drug dissolution, improve intestinal epithelial permeability and increment the permeability of tight junction. Surfactant in the formulation assumes a prevalent function to expand the retention of lipophilic drugs [18].

Co-surfactants

Various co-surfactants are utilized in these preparations such as alcohols and polyols of ethanol, isopropanol, butanol, benzyl alcohol, ethylene glycol, PG, butanediols and isomers thereof, glycerol, dimethyl isosorbide, pentaerythritol, sorbitol, polypropylene glycol, mannitol, transcutol, HPMC and other cellulosic polymers, cyclodextrins and its derivatives. Esters of PGs 200 to 6000 such as tetrahydrofuryl alcohol and PEG ether (glycofural) are utilized.

Amides of 2-pyrrlodone, 2-piperidone, N-alkylpiperidone, caprolactum, N-hydroxyalkyle pyrrolidone, N-alkylpyrrolidone, N-alkylcaprolactam and dimethylacetamide PVP are also employed.

Esters of ethyl propionate, tributyl citrate, triacetin, acetyl triethyle citrate, ethylene oleate, ethyl caprylate, ethyl butyrate, caprolactone, butyrolactone, propylene glycol diacetate, acetyl tributyl citrate, propylene glycol monoacetate, and valerolactone can also be employed [19].

The most commonly used co-solvents in SMEDDS are shown in Table **3**.

Table 3. Some examples of co-solvents commonly employed ingredients in SMEDDS.

S. No.	Marketed Name	Chemical Name	Regulatory Status
1.	Ethanol	-	Oral product, EP, USP-NF
3.	Transcutol P	Diethylene glycol monoethyl ether	EP, FDA IIG PG
3.	PEG	PEG 300 and PEG 400	Oral product, EP, USP-NF
4.	Glycerin	-	Oral product, EP, USP-NF

Various surfactants, co-surfactants and oils utilized for commercial purposes of LBFs are given in Table **4** [20, 21].

Table 4. Examples of surfactants, co-surfactants and oils utilized for commercial purposes of LBFs.

Commercial Name of the Ingredient	Commercially Available Products
Surfactants/co-surfactants	
Tween 20	Targretin soft gelatin capsule (SGC)
Tween 80	Gengraf hard gelatin capsule (HGC)
Span 80	Gengraf HGC
Cremophor EL	Gengraf HGC, Ritonavir oral solution

Commercial Name of the Ingredient	Commercially Available Products
Cremophor RH40	Neoral SGC, Ritonavir oral solution
Labrafil M 2125Cs	Sandimmune SGC
Labrafil M 1944Cs)	Sandimmune oral solution
D-α-Tocopheryl polyethylene glycol 1000 succinate	Agenerase SGC and its oral solution
Co-solvents	
Glycerin	Neoral SGC, Sandimmune SGC
Ethanol	Neoral SGC, Neoral oral solution, Gengraf HGC, Sandimmune SGC and oral solution
PG	Neoral SGC, Neoral oral solution, Lamprene SGC, Agenerase SGC, Agenerase oral solution, Gengraf HGC, Targretin SGC, Gengraf HGC, Agenerase SGC and its oral solution
Oils	
Corn oil mono-, di-, tri-glyceride	Neoral SGC and oral solution
DL-α-Tocopherol	Neoral oral solution, Fortovase SGC
Fractionated triglyceride of coconut oil (MCT)	Rocaltrol SGC, Hectorol SGC
Fractionated triglyceride of palm seed oil (MCT)	Rocaltrol oral solution
A mixture of mono- and di-glycerides of caprylic/capric acid	Avodart SGC
Medium-chain mono- and di-glycerides	Fortovase SGC
Corn oil	Sandimmune SGC, Depakene capsules
Olive oil	Sandimmune oral solution
Oleic acid	Ritonavir SGC, Norvir SGC
Sesame oil	Marinol SGC
Hydrogenated soybean oil	Accutane SGC, Vesanoid SGC
Cremophor	Accutane SGC, Vesanoid SGC
Soybean oil	Accutane SGC
Peanut oil	Prometrium SGC
Beeswax	Vesanoid SGC, Accutane SGC, Prometrium SGC

Other Components

Other components include pH adjusters, flavors and antioxidants. Auto-oxidation occurs due to the presence of lipid peroxides that boosts the unsaturation level of the lipid. So, lipid-soluble antioxidants may be required such as α-tocopherol, β-carotene propyl gallate, ascorbyl palmitate, or butyl hydroxyl toluene and butyl hydroxyl anisole, that could potentially be added in formulations to shield either unsaturated FA chains or drugs from oxidation [16].

Consistency Builder

Beeswax, cetyl alcohol can be incorporated to change the consistency of the emulsion.

Enzyme Inhibitors

Enzyme inhibitors can be incorporated into SMEDDS if the drug is prone to enzymatic degradation. For example, amino acids and modified amino acids such as amino-borinine derivatives [22].

IMPACT OF INGREDIENTS ON GLOBULES SIZE

The chain lengths of lipids have a significant effect on the globule size of SNEDDS in fasting state media. SNEDDS have 40% glycerides created the least globule size when formulation contains LC and MC glycerides. A comparative impact of unsaturated fat chain length on globule measure was seen by Thomas *et al.* [23].

MC glycerides are better to prepare fine droplets than LC glycerides since shorter FAs chains relate to greater hydrophilicity. Expanding MC glyceride concentrations from 40-75% brought about a bigger size of droplets. All emulsions created by MC, SNEDDS are anticipated to be monodisperse with average globule size less than 200 nm. The impact of LC glyceride concentration on globule size of emulsion was not explored on the grounds that LC6 with the least researched LC glyceride centralization of (40%) effectively created a polydisperse emulsion [24].

MULTI-FUNCTIONAL EXCIPIENT USED IN SEDDS/SMEDDS

Rice germ oil (RGO) is used as a multi-functional excipient in SEDDS. The RGO is obtained from *Oryza sativa* family Gramineae. RGO is an edible oil having 2.35:1.36:1 proportion of monounsaturated, polyunsaturated and saturated fatty acids, respectively. It consists of triglycerides, mainly C16–C18 fatty acids (81.3–84.3% w/w). RGO is one of the richest sources of potent antioxidant gamma-oryzanol (4–5% w/w). Gamma oryzanol is ferulic acid ester derivatives such as 10-phytosteryl ferulates, cycloartenyl ferulate, 24-methylenecycloartanyl ferulate and campesteryl ferulate. It has various medicinal applications such as prevention of cancer, maintenance of plasma lipid level and prevention of platelet aggregation. An accelerated oxidation study demonstrated the capability of gamma-oryzanol in preventing lipid peroxidation of oils. Tacrolimus (TAC) is a macrolide antibiotic having potent immunosuppressant activity with very short and variable bioavailability due to its poor solubility, first-pass metabolism and inter-subject variability [17].

Hence, Pawar *et al.,* 2012 prepared the SMEDDS of TAC using gamma-oryzano--enriched RGO as a multi-functional excipient having inherent antioxidant potential as well as higher solubilization capacity for lipophilic drugs like TAC [25].

HLB VALUE ICI established a systematic design of centering down on the relatively few emulsifiers appropriate for any specified purpose to save time in the selection of emulsifiers, which is known as the HLB system.

Relation of HLB with the Solubility

The HLB and solubility of an emulsifier are correlated to each other. Thus, an emulsifier that has less HLB has a solubility in oil and one having a greater HLB has a solubility in water.

Requirement of HLB- Why HLB Required?

The HLB system is used for the prediction of the optimum emulsifying stability. When the HLB value of the surfactant is equivalent with required HLB, then it results in development of the o/w or w/o type emulsion system. Process optimization can be attained by only incorporating surfactant frameworks with the same HLB value.

The huge number of surfactants are present, coupled with the truth that their usage troubles are increasing, which creates the requirement for the choice of appropriate surfactants.

HLB Calculation

From viewpoints of product quality and yield, the determination of HLB value of a surfactant is very important that can be calculated theoretically or experimentally. In 1949, William Griffin described the experimental technique for calculating HLB value experimentally [26 - 30].

CONSENT FOR PUBLICATION

Not applicable.

CONFLICT OF INTEREST

The author declares no conflict of interest, financial or otherwise.

ACKNOWLEDGEMENTS

Declared none.

REFERENCES

[1]   Gupta S, Kesarla R, Omri A. Formulation strategies to improve the bioavailability of poorly absorbed drugs with special emphasis on self-emulsifying systems. ISRN Pharm 2013; 2013848043
[http://dx.doi.org/10.1155/2013/848043] [PMID: 24459591]

[2]   Tejeswari N, Harini CV, Hyndavi N, Jyotsna T, Gowri Y, Raju YP. Lipid-based drug delivery system for enhancing oral bioavailability–a contemporary review. J Glob Trends Pharm Sci 2014; 5(4): 2074-82.

[3]   Yetukuri K, Sudheer P. Approaches to development of solid-self micron emulsifying drug delivery system: Formulation techniques and dosage forms: A review. Int J Pharm Sci Res 2012; 3(10): 3550-63.

[4]   Parmar B, Patel U, Bhimani B, Sanghavi K, Patel G, Daslaniya D. SMEDDS: A dominant dosage form which improve bioavailability. Am J Pharm Tech Res 2012; 2(4): 54-72.

[5]   Prachi S, Prajapati SK, Shipra S, Ali A. A review on SMEDDS: An approach to enhance oral bioavailability of poorly water-soluble drugs. Int Res J Pharm 2016; 4(7): 1-6.

[6]   Nigade PM, Patil SL, Tiwari SS. Self-emulsifying drug delivery system (SEDDS): A review. Int J Pharma Bio Sci 2012; 2(2): 42-52.

[7]   Nikolakakis I, Malamataris S. Self-emulsifying pellets: relations between kinetic parameters of drug release and emulsion reconstitution-influence of formulation variables. J Pharm Sci 2014; 103(5): 1453-65.
[http://dx.doi.org/10.1002/jps.23919] [PMID: 24596121]

[8]   Mu H, Holm R, Müllertz A. Lipid-based formulations for oral administration of poorly water-soluble drugs. Int J Pharm 2013; 453(1): 215-24.
[http://dx.doi.org/10.1016/j.ijpharm.2013.03.054] [PMID: 23578826]

[9]   Muchow M, Maincent P, Müller RH. Lipid nanoparticles with a solid matrix (SLN, NLC, LDC) for oral drug delivery. Drug Dev Ind Pharm 2008; 34(12): 1394-405.
[http://dx.doi.org/10.1080/03639040802130061] [PMID: 18665980]

[10]   Pouton CW, Porter CJ. Formulation of lipid-based delivery systems for oral administration: materials, methods and strategies. Adv Drug Deliv Rev 2008; 60(6): 625-37.
[http://dx.doi.org/10.1016/j.addr.2007.10.010] [PMID: 18068260]

[11]   Verma R, Mittal V, Kaushik D. Self-microemulsifying drug delivery system: A vital approach for bioavailability enhancement. Int J Chemtech Res 2017; 10(7): 515-28.

[12]   Müller RH, Mäder K, Gohla S. Solid lipid nanoparticles (SLN) for controlled drug delivery - a review of the state of the art. Eur J Pharm Biopharm 2000; 50(1): 161-77.
[http://dx.doi.org/10.1016/S0939-6411(00)00087-4] [PMID: 10840199]

[13]   Ramya A, Sudheer P, Sogali BS. Self-emulsifying drug delivery system-an innovative approach for enhancement of solubility and therapeutic potential. J Pharma Res 2016; 15(4): 153-61.
[http://dx.doi.org/10.18579/jpcrkc/2016/15/4/108824]

[14]   Chaus HA, Chopade VV, Chaudhri PD. Self-emulsifying drug delivery system: A review. Int J Pharm Chem Sci 2013; 2(4): 34-44.

[15] Verma R, Kaushik D. Design and optimization of candesartan loaded self-nanoemulsifying drug delivery system for improving its dissolution rate and pharmacodynamic potential 2020.

[16] Zhang Y, Wang R, Wu J, Shen Q. Characterization and evaluation of self-microemulsifying sustained-release pellet formulation of puerarin for oral delivery. Int J Pharm 2012; 427(2): 337-44. [http://dx.doi.org/10.1016/j.ijpharm.2012.02.013] [PMID: 22366381]

[17] Wagh MP, Singh PK, Chaudhari CS, Khairnar DA. Solid self-emulsifying drug delivery system: Preparation techniques and dosage forms. Int J Biopharm 2014; 5(2): 101-18.

[18] Khan A, Khan H, Mohamad T, Rasul A. Basics of SMEDDS. J Pharm and Alternative Med 2012; 4(9): 13-20.

[19] Shah I. Development and characterization of oil-in-water nanoemulsions from self-microemulsifying mixtures 2011.

[20] Mahapatra AK, Murthy PN, Swadeep B, Swain RP. Self-emulsifying drug delivery systems (SEDDS): An update from formulation development to therapeutic strategies. Int J Pharm Tech Res 2014; 6(2): 546-68.

[21] Sonia A, Gupta R. Self–micro emulsifying drug delivery system: A review. World J Pharm Pharm Sci 2015; 4(8): 502-22.

[22] Deokate UA, Shinde NI, Bhingare UJ. Novel approaches for development and characterization of SMEDDS. Int J Curr Pharm Res 2013; 5(4): 5-12.

[23] Thomas N, Müllertz A, Graf A, Rades T. Influence of lipid composition and drug load on the *In Vitro* performance of self-nanoemulsifying drug delivery systems. J Pharm Sci 2012; 101(5): 1721-31. [http://dx.doi.org/10.1002/jps.23054] [PMID: 22294458]

[24] Tran T, Xi X, Rades T, Müllertz A. Formulation and characterization of self-nanoemulsifying drug delivery systems containing monoacyl phosphatidylcholine. Int J Pharm 2016; 502(1-2): 151-60. [http://dx.doi.org/10.1016/j.ijpharm.2016.02.026] [PMID: 26915809]

[25] Pawar SK, Vavia PR. Rice germ oil as multifunctional excipient in preparation of self-microemulsifying drug delivery system (SMEDDS) of tacrolimus. AAPS PharmSciTech 2012; 13(1): 254-61. [http://dx.doi.org/10.1208/s12249-011-9748-1] [PMID: 22232022]

[26] Khadka P, Ro J, Kim H, *et al.* Pharmaceutical particle technologies: An approach to improve drug solubility, dissolution and bioavailability. Asian J Pharm Sci 2014; 9(6): 304-16. [http://dx.doi.org/10.1016/j.ajps.2014.05.005]

[27] Thakare P, Mogal V, Borase P, Dusane J, Kshirsagar S. A review on self-emulsified drug delivery system. J Pharm Biolog Evalu 2016; 3(2): 140-53.

[28] Zhang L, Zhang L, Zhang M, *et al.* Self-emulsifying drug delivery system and the applications in herbal drugs. Drug Deliv 2015; 22(4): 475-86. [http://dx.doi.org/10.3109/10717544.2013.861659] [PMID: 24321014]

[29] Agarwal V, Alayoubi A, Siddiqui A, Nazzal S. Powdered self-emulsified lipid formulations of meloxicam as solid dosage forms for oral administration. Drug Dev Ind Pharm 2012; 3(4): 1-9. [PMID: 23072611]

[30] Solans C, Izquierdo P, Nolla J. Nano-emulsions. Curr Opin Colloid Interface Sci 2005; 10: 102-10. [http://dx.doi.org/10.1016/j.cocis.2005.06.004]

CHAPTER 5

Lymphatic Transport of Lipid-Based Drug Delivery System

Ravinder Verma[1], Deepak Kaushik[1,*], Beena Kumari[2] and Anurag Khatkar[1]

[1] *Department of Pharmaceutical Sciences, Maharshi Dayanand University, Rohtak (Haryana), 124001, India*

[2] *Department of Pharmaceutical Sciences, Indra Gandhi University, Meerpur, Rewari, India*

Abstract: The gastrointestinal tract is abundantly provided with both lymphatic and blood vessels. In this way, material or drugs that are retained over the small intestinal epithelial cells can conceivably go through either lymphatic or blood vessels. The larger parts of drugs or compounds are transported into blood vessels because of a high flow rate (500-overlay), greater than that of intestinal lymph. Lymphatic transport of drugs will occur when the drug is profoundly lipophilic (log P >5) and demonstrates high solubility in TGs (>50mg/ml). Type of lipid, co-administered lipid substance, and level of unsaturation of lipid can alter the degree of lymphatic drug transportation. Biopharmaceutical issues such as increment in the rate of disintegration and dissolvability in the intestinal fluids, shieldthe drug from chemical and enzymatic degradation in the oil globules. The development of lipoproteins favor lymphatic transportation of highly hydrophobic drugs. The food impact is gathered throughout the ongoing decades, and it depends on the various components emerging from physiology, dosage form, and physicochemical features. The dietary lipids that occur in the food also play a role as solubilizers for drugs and consequently experience the lipid digestion by gastric and pancreatic lipases, similar to the mechanism depicted for LBFs to create different micellar species. A variety of *in vitro* models can act as a substitute to *in vivo* models for the investigation of lymphatic drug transport. In the intestinal permeability model, caco-2 cells are utilized to estimate the intracellular lipoprotein-lipid assembly. Animal models are used to investigate the direct estimation of the drug *via* lymphatic drug transport by cannulation of the intestinal lymphatic duct. Rat is mainly used as an animal model, but other large animals such as dogs, pigs, and sheep have also been reported. Most SMEDDS formulations have not been capable to come into the sale due to lack of effective *in vitro* tests that are representative of authentic *in vivo* behavior. Impact of lipidic excipients, the influence of self-emulsifying lipid-based formulations on food effect, and reduction of food effect are discussed thoroughly; these affect limited lymphatic assimilation. This chapter highlights the

* **Corresponding author Deepak Kaushik:** Department of Pharmaceutical Sciences, Maharshi Dayanand University, Rohtak (Haryana), 124001, India; Tel: +91 9315809626;
E-mail: deepkaushik1977@gmail.com

various lymphatic mechanisms that help in attaining improved bioavailability, various factors, and various models used for the assessment of drug assimilation *via* the lymphatic system.

Keywords: Animal model for lymphatic transport, Food effect, Intestinal transportation, Lipid solubility, Lipoproteins, Lymphatic system.

LYMPHATIC TRANSPORT

The lymphatic system of our body is an element of the circulatory system that is composed of a complicated system of ducts consisting of a clear fluid known as lymph. Their main role is holding extracellular fluid and keeping the balance of body water. The interstitial space leaks out extracellular fluid back to the blood circulation that helps in the maintenance of body water [1, 2]. Furthermore, it has a specialized function at particular sites due to its non-uniform structure and function all over the body. It also helps in the assimilation of cholesterol esters, long-chain fatty acids (LCFAs), lipid-soluble vitamins, triglycerides (TGs), and xenobiotics [3]. Drug delivery through this system has numerous benefits that include bypassing the first-pass metabolism and target specific drugs for ailments that spread *via* this system, such as specific types of tumors and HIV. It plays an active role in the distribution of metastatic tumor cells. Tumor cells utilize the lymph nodes, which act as a reservoir for these cells to spread to other regions of the body [4].

There is an increase in the number of hydrophobic drugs, which resulted in the development of various formulation approaches to aid the assimilation of drugs with low aqueous solubility and high lipophilicity. Both lymphatic and blood vessels occur in a huge amount in GIT, resulting in the assimilation of drugs over the small intestinal (SI) epithelial cells either *via* lymphatic or blood vessels. Most of the drugs are uptaken into blood vessels because of a higher flow rate (500-times) than intestinal lymph. Lymphatic transport of drugs will occur when the drug is profoundly lipophilic (logP >5) and demonstrates high solubility in TGs (> 50 mg/ml). These drugs are assimilated through lymph vessels in the intestine *via* conjugation with created lipoproteins (LPs) in the enterocyte. These LPs transport druf to the lymphatic entrance that is responsible for retention of lipids. They avoid liver metabolism because of drugs transported by the lymph vessels [5].

Transportation of drugs *via* the intestinal lymphatic vessels occurs by three mechanisms [6]. Firstly, through lymphatic capillaries, which consist of single-layered, non-fenestrated endothelial cells that are arranged in a highly gapped and overlapped manner to shape a porous partition in the lymphatic vasculature. This feature permits macromolecular targeting to the lymphatic system. Hence, an absorption enhancer can be used to enhance the assimilation of these compounds, which is feasible by opening up the paracellular route. Secondly, gut-associated lymphoid tissue contains peyer's patches (isolated or aggregated lymphoid follicles) that helps in the entry of drugs into the lymphatic system [7 - 10]. Transcellular absorption, paracellular transport, P-gp, and cytochrome P450 inhibition pathways are used by intestinal walls to transport lipids, which is the primary route. Enhanced generation of chylomicrons is linked with the delivery of hydrophobic candidates into the lymphatic system [11].

Several LBFs such as emulsion (penclomedine, ontazolast), microemulsion (puerarin, raloxifene), micellar systems (cyclosporin A), SEEDS (coenzyme Q10), SMEDDS (halofantrine, valsartan, nobiletin, sirolimus, vinpocetine, silymarin) SNEDDS (valsartan, carvedilol, halofantrine), liposomes (IgGI, doxorubicin, cefotaxime, 9-nitro-camptothecin, paclitaxel, ovalbumin) SLNs (etoposide, methotrexate, idarubicin, tobramycin, nimodipine), NLCs (testosterone, vinpocetine, tripterine), *etc.* have been examined for the lymphatic transport [12 - 43].

BENEFITS

1. It provides safety of drugs from the first-pass metabolism by evading first pass through the liver that is responsible for improvement in oral bioavailability of formulation.

2. They can be intended for target-specific drug formulation.

3. They can change the toxicological profiles of the formulation.

Approaches to Upgrade Lymphatic Transportation of the Drug

Drug transportation across intestinal lymph relies on the drug association with generated lipoproteins (LPs) in enterocytes. The association of drug and lipoprotein is the primary key to improve lymphatic transportation of drugs. Type of lipid, co-administered lipid substance, and the level of unsaturation of lipid can alter the degree of lymphatic drug transportation. Prodrug strategy may improve the lymphatic transport of the drugs by means of covalent coupling of drugs to lipidic contents such as FA, DGs, or phosphoglyceride.

Favorable Circumstances of Intestinal Transportation of Drugs

Due to the extraordinary life systems and physiology of lymphatics, intestinal lymphatic drug transportation can give various focal points over drug retention through the blood.

The GIT is lavishly provided with both lymphatics and veins. In this way, materials that are ingested over the SI epithelial cells can enter either blood vessels or lymphatics. The dominant parts of consumed materials are transported into the blood because the rate of flow in the blood is roughly 500-overlay greater than that of intestinal lymph. Highly lipophilic drugs may, in this way, get to the intestinal lymph through creating LPs in the enterocyte.

In any case, where easy dissemination over the blood slim endothelium is constrained, for instance, high atomic weight, the specific transportation into intestinal lymph may exist because the lymphatic vessels have more porosity than neighboring blood vessels. Ingestion of high molecular weight drug takes pace into the enterocyte and then drug enter into the intestinal lymph because of post-absorptive relationship with colloidal LPs amid transportation through the enterocyte.

The recognizable proof of progressively lipophilic drug has managed a current increment in enthusiasm for the components by which drugs get to the lymph, the formulation strategies that might be considered to augment or limit lymphatic transportation and the possible effect of lymphatic transportation on drug both inside enterocyte and liver. Lymphatic transportation has appeared to be a supporter of improved oral bioavailability of several exceptionally hydrophobic drugs and different xenobiotics after ingesting orally. It includes various drugs such as cannabinoids, halofantrine, moxidectin, mepitiostane, testosterone subordinates, MK-386, penclomedine, naftifine, probucol, cyclosporine, ontazolast, benzopyrene, polychlorinated biphenyls and various hydrophobic prodrugs. Conversely, just little amounts of more hydrophilic drugs such as salicylic acid, isoniazid and caffeine are recouped in lymph after ingesting orally.

For instance, the drugs that are ingested through this route are shielded from gastric first-pass digestion since mesenteric lymph opposes the entry of the blood For the drugs that are exceedingly metabolized on the first pass *via* the liver, their transport through this system can upgrade their oral bioavailability. Besides the essential course of metastatic spread of various tumors, this system is the fundamental transport pathway for B and T lymphocytes. Thusly, it has been recommended that immunomodulatory and anticancer mixes might be more viable when ingested through lymphatic transport [44].

Parameters Affecting Lymphatic Transportation of LBFs

Compounds or drug moieties such as antitumor, anti-HIV and immunosuppressive agents are GI sensitive. That is why they have been formulated into LBFs. LBFs are assimilated and distributed *via* the GI epithelium to the peripheral lymphatic duct that has been investigated [45]. Several researchers researched the lymphatic system have found that assimilation of LBFs and their distribution in this system is relying on the route of administrating, size of globule, charge on surface, molecular weight, lipophilicity, kind of lipid and emulsifier´s concentration. This has also been described in detail below and shown in Fig. (**1**) [46].

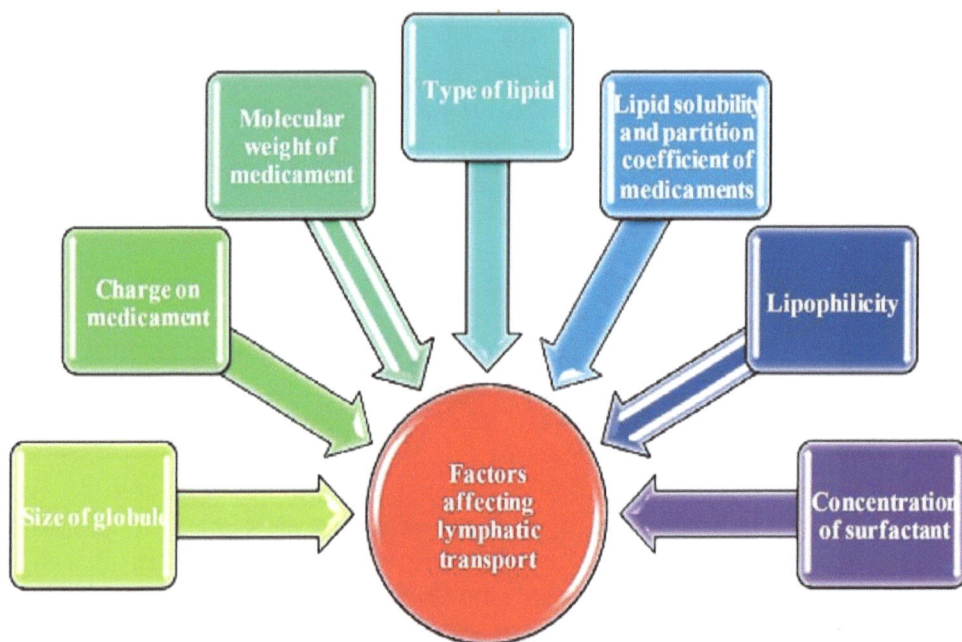

Fig. (1). Various factors affecting lymphatic transport.

Size of Globules

Lymphatic uptake and assimilation in lymph nodes depend on the size and composition of LBFs. Various drug candidates such as monoclonal antibodies and antineoplastic agents are formulated as dendrimers and LBFs, based on the nature of the formulation for specifically targeting the lymphatic system [47]. Oussoren *et al.,* reported that 10–100 nm is the most selected particle size for lymphatic assimilation *via s/c* route [48]. If globule size is less than 10 nm then, it is assimilated through the blood circulation, while globule size >100 nm demonstrates superior assimilation through this system but at a slow rate. Still, globules having a size greater than 100 nm have not been defined. Additionally, the scientists found that if the interstitial injection of particles greater than 100 nm is administered gradually, then formulation remained at the administration site for a specific time duration.

Charge on Drug

Zeta potential is an essential parameter in the lymphatic assimilation of drugs. It has been found that some anionic carriers such as dendrimers, nanospheres and lipid-based nanoparticles demonstrated greater lymphatic uptake than cationic or neutral charged carriers because of the anionic nature of the interstitial matrix [49]. So, in the interstitial matrix, anionic carrier encoun-ters electrostatic repulsion and shift more hastily [11]. Highly anionic particles are found to be kept for a long duration in lymph nodes [50]. On the other hand, cationic charged carriers in the interstitium face greater opposition to travel to the -vely charged interstitium matrix due to enhancement of electrostatic attractive force. Information related to the ionic nature of carrier molecules is obtained through zeta potential. Zeta potential of -30 mV shows an intensely anionic nature, values in the range of +10 to -10 mV specify neutral charge and +30 mV values show- a cationic nature [51].

Kaur *et al.,* investigated zidovudine loaded liposomes embodied with either cationic (stearylamine) or anionic (*i.e.* dicetyl phosphate) charge surfactants to target the lymphatic system. Liposomal transportation *via* lymph is identified by fluorescent microscopy and they concluded that the anionic charged liposomes enhanced lymphatic uptake in contrast to cationic liposomes [52]. One more investigation, conducted by Patel *et al.,* found that by the lymph nodes, the sequence of liposomal assimilation to be as: anionic > cationic > neutral charge [53].

Molecular Weight of Drug

A linear relationship is obtained among molecular weight and assimilation rate of macromolecules *via* subcutaneous route through lymphatic drug delivery. An increment in the molecular weight decreases uptake of compounds by capillaries and improves uptake at the injection site into the lymphatic system. Drugs that have molecular weight >1000 Daltons are without difficulty assimilated by the capillaries prior to their entry into the lymphatic circulation. While, drugs having a molecular weight of more than 16,000 Daltons have a propensity to be assimilated by this system rather than by the capillaries [46].

Lipophilicity

Hawley *et al.,* demonstrated that lipophilicity assists in the facilitation of lymphatic uptake of LBFs from the site of administration [54]. The lipophilicity of the molecules is associated with their surface features and primarily liable for phagocytosis and their lymphatic uptake. As the lipophilicity of bacteria decreases, phagocytosis increases opsonization due to attachment of opsonins more effortlessly to lipophilic surfaces than to hydrophilic surfaces, concluded Dahlback *et al.* This will result in an increase in phagocytosis and thus improvement of lymphatic uptake [55].

Lipid Solubility and Partition Coefficient of Drugs

Physicochemical features such as lipid solubility and partition coefficient of drugs play an important role in the lymphatic transportation of drugs. Charman and Stella found that TG solubility (>50 mg/ml) and the log P value (>5) of a candidate are required for effective lymphatic transport [56]. They judge lymphatic transportation of dichlorodiphenyl-trichloroethane (log P 6.19) and log P 6.53 of hexachlorobenzene. The log P values of both drugs are identical, but they have dissimilarity in TG solubility, with dichlorodiphenyltrichloroe-thane having 13-times higher TG solubility than hexachlorobenzene. It was concluded that dichlorodiphenyltrichloro-ethane had greater lymphatic uptake (33.5%) compared to hexachlorobenzene (2.3%). They summarized that this variation in lymphatic trans¬port may exist because of TG solubility variation in these drugs. On the other hand, Myers and Stella found that greater log P value and high lipid solubility did not result in considerable lymphatic uptake at all times such as Penclomedine having log P (5.48) and lipid solubility (175 mg/ml) resulted in poor lymphatic uptake (only about 3%). This may be because of the lesser affinity of this drug for chylomicrons than RBCs and plasma proteins, that resulted in its higher concentrations of blood than lymph [12].

Type of Lipid

Fundamentally, LBFs consist of TGs that organize themselves in a manner that the polar head is out to the aqueous medium identical to the arrangement of chylomicrons. Assimilation of lipids *via* transcellular route through polar intestinal epithelial cells may be affected by lipid composition in the formulation. Paliwal *et al.*, formulated methotrexate-loaded SLNs with four types of lipidic ingredients such as stearic acid, compritol 888 ATO, monostearin and tristearin by using the solvent diffusion method and evaluated them based on their globule charge, morphology, size, entrapment of drug, *in vitro* discharge and pharmacokinetic properties. SLNs having compritol 888 ATO showed the highest entrapment efficiency and minimum size. The benefits of compritol 888 ATO over other lipidic ingredients could be because of glyceryl behenate long-chain, which offers the interchain insertion site for methotrexate molecule,. That why researchers found that SLNs had improved bioavailability than others. An anesthetized albino rat model was used for *in situ* investigation to assess lymphatic uptake through cannulation of the mesenteric duct. The lymphatic drug amount profile illustrated that this preparation had maximum lymphatic uptake in comparison to other preparations. Furthermore, the researchers found a correlation among their *in vitro* and *in situ* outcomes [57].

Concentration of Surfactant

The concentration of the surfactant directly affects the partitioning of a drug in LBFs. Thus, it can indirectly affect the release of the drug at the targetted site. Sanjula *et al.,* formulated carvedilol SLNs with 5%-15% poloxamer 188 (surfactant) and investigated the impact of range of concentrations of surfactant on lymphatic uptake and entrapment efficiency. They observed that an increment in their con¬centration resulted in a diminishment of the entrapment efficiency which may be because of production of micelles of poloxamer 188 at higher concentrations that resulted in an increase in the solubility of carvedilol in the aqueous phase and resulted in lesser drug entrapment. Similar results were obtained after *in vivo* study that was executed in male Wistar rats [58].

VARIOUS MODELS UTILIZED FOR INVESTIGATION OF DRUG TRANSPORTATION *VIA* LYMPHATIC SYSTEM

Models for *In Vivo*

In this model, cannulation of the thoracic or mesenteric lymphatic ducts is done in animals to study drug transportation in the intestinal lymphatic system [59]. The *in vivo* model permits for direct assessment of drug amount in lymph. This method cannot be executed on humans due to the irreversible and invasive surgical process. Small animals (mice and rats) are usually used, but sometimes bigger animals such as rabbits, sheep, dogs, pigs, *etc.* are also used for these models [60].

The lymphatic venous shunt is another *in vivo* model in which drug concentrations are calculated at a predetermined time in lymph and lymph is collected over an extended time. In an oral bioavailability investigation, an indirect method is used to assess the intestinal lymphatic drug transportation in both presence and absence of inhibitors of intestinal chylomicron flow. No involvement of a surgry, as occurs in the lymphatic duct cannulation model is the benefit of this method [61 - 64].

Models for *In Vitro*

A variety of *in vitro* models can act as a substitute to *in vivo* models for the investigation of lymphatic drug transport. Caco-2 cells are utilized in the intestinal permeability model to estimate intracellular lipoprotein-lipid assembly and study the effect of lipid and lipidic ingredients on the addition of drugs with LPs in lymphatic transport [65 - 67]. Gershkovich and Hoffman *et al.,* illustrated a correlation between the degree of *ex vivo* incorporation of a drug into chylomicrons and the amount of intestinal lymphatic drug transport in one *in vitro* model [68]. According to Dahan and Hoffman, *in vivo* drug assimilation could be forecasted by estimating the drug discharge from LBFs and estimating precipitation of the drug amid lipolysis [61]. Holm and Hoest *et al.,* found in silico technique that can recognize a quantitative correlation among molecular structure and quantity of drug transported from this system [69].

Evaluation of Animal Model for Lymphatic Transport

Animal models are used to investigate the direct estimation of drugs *via* lymphatic drug passage using cannulation of the intestinal lymphatic duct. The primary animal model utilized are rats but some other animals like sheep, dogs and pigs have been reported. With a variety of modifications in the feeding and rehydration, the site of cannulation, pre- and postoperative methods, lymph fistulation and dosing, the rat model is widely used in different investigations [70].

In brief, a triple-cannulation of carotid artery (systemic blood collection), mesenteric lymph duct (intestinal lymph collection) and the duodenum (administering rehydration solution) is executed. However, it can also consist of a fourth cannula in the jugular vein if i/v administration is essential.

The mesenteric lymph cannula permits the withdrawal of all lymph draining to the duodenum and as a result, the total amount of drug transported by this system can be estimated [71].

The systemic blood collected from the carotid artery permits the estimation of blood plasma exposure that can be considered as the assimilation of the drug through systemic circulation. This method or model is valuable since it permits the evaluation of portal blood assimilation contribution to bioavailability by contrasting plasma exposure of orally administered drug with lymph duct cannulated rats and with plasma exposure of intravenously administered drug that are not lymph duct cannulated rats. Although, as expected in any animal model that with cannulation, the most general hurdle can be occlusion of the cannula [60, 62]. It makes the method deadly and complicates to employ.

In recent times, using colchicines, intestinal chylomicron flow inhibitors and Pluronic-L81 are some of the indirect pharmacological methods. In this method, blood drug contact is compared in the existence and absence of co-ingested Pluronic-L81 to indirectly evaluate the impact of intestinal lymphatic drug transportation in bioavailability. This method is beneficial as it does not need a lymph duct cannulation. Yet, in lipid processing, the effect of blocking chylomicron flow and synthesis has to be entirely described. For example, Pluronic-L81 lessens plasma VLDL, LDL and cholesterol levels in plasma and declines secretion of lipid and apoprotein [72]. Hyaluronic acid is a biocompatible polymer that follows lymphatic drainage from the interstitial spaces. A cis-platin hyaluronic acid conjugate was designed for intra-lymphatic deliverance of drugs [73].

To get better contrast in various in MRI imaging,various nanoparticles have been formulated consisting of gadolinium-based agents (gadolinium-diethylenetriamine penta-acetic acid) and iron oxide [74]. However, the use of cannulae is still the most frequently used method in animal modeling.

Lack of Effective *In Vitro* Tests

Most of SMEDDS products have not been capable to come into the sale because of the absence of efficient *in vitro* tests that are representative of authentic *in vivo* behavior. The performance of LBFs varies quite definitely among varying physiological milieu because their performance considerably relies on in situ parameters [75]. In some cases, *in vitro* dissolution can be employed as a surrogate indicator of *in vivo* dissolution [76]. The simple buffer media utilized for evaluation of the dissolution profile of PWS drugs is often narrow because of troube in attaining sink conditions.

Issues of sink condition can be defeated by the incorporation of surfactants/co-surfactants in dissolution media [77]. The dissolution media should be able to mimic the solubilization process of *in vivo* conditions to get better precision of *in vivo* dissolution results. The composition of numerous dissolution media has been modified mainly on similar levels of endogenous BS and PLs in fasting and fed conditions. For non-ionizable drugs, a good relationship is obtained among dissolution profiles of simulated fasting-state and fed-state intestinal media. For candidates over the similar physiological range with appreciable ionization, the condition is problematic due to the influence of both solubilization and ionization on solubility [78].

LIMITED LYMPHATIC UPTAKE OF LBDDS

A combination of fluid and protein, squeezed out of the blood that has been filtered is known as lymph. Lymphatic transport *via* the intestine has been established to be an assimilation pathway for hydrophobic drugs through the oral route. Hydrophobic drugs diffuse through intestinal enterocytes linked with secretable enterocyte LP chylomicron. Bone marrow, lymph nodes, spleen and thymus gland are interconnected with the lymph organs by lymph ducts [63, 79].

Lymphatic capillaries play an important function in the assimilation of particulate and their lymphatic assimilation.

For targeted deliverance, chylomicrons are the carrier systems that consist of triacylglycerols. Drug associates with it and secretes drug from enterocyte into lymphatic circulation despite blood circulation and candidates in intestinal lymph achieve contacts to blood circulation at the joint of subclavian veins and left internal jugular.

The first-pass metabolism bypasses when drugs are conveyed lymphatically. As a result, the concentration of drug and duration action increases. Alternatively, from alimentary canal hepatic portal system starts and it terminates in the liver. Drugs that pass through the hepatic portal system reach the liver before reaching systemic circulation where their first pass metabolism occurs.

The normal lymph flow in 24 hrs is 2-4 liter [80]. The ratio estimated 500:1 is for lymph flow *versus* blood flow, thus in the cases where targeting strategy is not adopted, most drugs diverted to the blood system.

A thin layer of non-fenestrated endothelial cells forms the walls of the capillary lymphatic that are widely overlapped and gapped, forming various pores and clefts [81]. These pores permit the transfer of macromolecules into the capillary lumen. 10-80 nm is an optimum range for lymphatic uptake of subcutaneously injected formulations while >100 nm will retain at the site of injection and minor particles are assimilated through the capillary framework that drains into the systemic circulation. When small neutral liposomes (>40 nm) were injected subcutaneously, <60–70% of those were cleared within 24 hours at the site of injection, only 30-40% of the dose were left at the injection site. On the other hand, liposomes having globule size of <500 nm are retained 60-80% at the site of injection [82]. Thus, nanocarriers administered subcutaneously have more potential for delivering antineoplastic agents to lymphatic metastases.

Lymphatic transportation has been established to be more efficient for immunomodulatory and chemotherapeutic drugs because it is the main route for transport pathway for T and B lymphocytes and metastasis of solid tumors. The spreading of HIV, hepatitis B and C virus, morbillivirus and various acute respiratory syndrome-related coronavirus are linked with lymphocytes present in lymphoid tissue and lymph.

Oral intake of various types of TGs (LCT, MCT and SCT) to the lymph cannulated fasted rat was investigated. The quantity of LCT present in the lymph was found to be 3-9 times greater than MCT and SCT. This may be because of the stimulatory effect on the secretion and lymphatic transportation of endogenous

LCT of exogenously administered LCT.

The impact is hypothesized to lessen with a decline in the chain length of exogenously administered TG, *i.e.* LCT > MCT > SCT [83]. Comparatively, even a small amount of LCT can stimulate contraction of the gall bladder and result in the increased levels of intestinal BS, PLs and cholesterol. The rate of this stimulatory response increases as the quantity of LCT administered improves. In contrast, the intake of the same amount of MCT established relatively low effects on the contraction of the gallbladder and did not stimulate a significant increment in the intestinal concentration of BS. Hence, FAs with MC length are transported mainly by the systemic circulation, whereas those with longer chain length are added primarily into chylomicrons and transported through lymph.

About 43.7% of halofantrine hydrochloride (Hf-HCl) transport dose occurs *via* lymphatic transportation after oral post-prandial administration to the dogs. More lipophilic free base is generated during lipolysis that gets associated with chylomicron and results in great lymphatic transport of Hf-HCl. High log P value and TGs solubility do not always give assurance of considerable lymphatic uptake [84].

In Vivo Studies based on Dispersed Formulations for Lymphatic Assimilation

Lymphatic drug transportation that depends on the content of GI lipid assimilation can contribute considerably to the overall assimilation of hydrophobic drugs from GIT. Since the effective assimilation of lipidic ingredients and co-solubilized lipophilic xenobiotics from GIT depends upon the early development of fine o/w dispersion, the impact of dispersion on lymphatic transportation has been examined. Porter *et al.,* got the same results of lymphatic transportation for assimilation of anti-malarial drug (halofantrine) after oral ingestion of micellar solution, an emulsion and a lipidic solution to mesenteric, in conscious lymph cannulated rats. However, while they repeat investigations with anesthetized rats in which GI motility and capability disperse the ingested lipid, the relative contribution of lymphatic uptake of halofantrine to overall drug assimilation was directly linked with the degree of lipid dispersion associated with ingested formulation [85].

The lymphotropic activity of ontazolast loaded SEDDS/SMEDDS preparations of the LTB4 biosynthesis inhibitor was investigated in conscious mesenteric lymph fistula rats [13]. Preparations consisting of 50:50 or 80:20 ratio concentrations of Gelucire 44/14 and Peceol, a solution in Peceol and an LCT emulsion, all offered the same increment in bioavailability of the drug in comparison to an aqueous suspension as a reference. SEDDS formulation assists the most quick drug assimilation in lymph whereas the LCT emulsion showed the greatest drug uptake in mesenteric lymph. These results recommended that SEDDS may have potential as lymphotropic delivery systems but there should be a balance between the concentrations of surfactants and lipidic ingredients, which helps in keeping the drug in the solution form in the GIT amid assimilation while lipidic substrate helps for the production of the chylomicrons. The same results were obtained by Ichihashi [86].

Impact of Lipidic Excipients on Lymphatic Transport

Halofantrine loaded SMEDDS consisting of either MCT or LCT as the lipidic ingredients has been investigated in conscious dogs for mesenteric lymphatic transport. The amount of ingested dose of Hf transported in the lymph was 28.3% after administration of the LC-SMEDDS while only 5% in the case of MC-SMEDDS by its contents of MGs and DGs of MCTs, which unlike LCFA, are not lymphotropic. A similar study was conducted by Holm et al. with SMEDDS in which MCT and LCT lipidic ingredients were interchanged with "structured TGs" [Medium long medium-chain fatty acids (MLM) and Long medium long-chain fatty acid (LML)]. Structured TGs are prepared by selective esterifying medium and LCFA to specific positions on the glycerol backbone of the TG molecule. MLM-SMEDDS of halofantrine enhanced 17.9% in contrast to MC-SMEDDS, but in the case of LML-SMEDDS was 27.4% which was similar to that of the LC-SMEDDS (28.3%). The apparent, better rate of transport of halofantrine was found for the structured lipid, MLM-SMEDDS in comparison to MC-SMEDDS due to high LCFA content of surfactant, maiscine 35-1 employed in MLM-SMEDDS to facilitate self-emulsification [18].

The other studies show the potential utility that SEDDS or SMEDDS formulation for the development of LBDDS. These outcomes emerge by the addition of ingredients containing LCT that favors synthesis of chylomicrons and by the enhancement of dispersion of these preparations in GIT, which seems to assist lymphatic drug transport by aiding digestion and assimilation of lipid.

Impact Food on Self-emulsification of LBFs

Elevation in drug exposure, relative to fasting condition, subsequent postprandial intake of PWS drugs in the conventional solid products is well reported in the literature (such as isotretinoin, danazol, DPC961, halofantrine). It has been hypothesized that an increment in the magnitude of the exposure may show the achievable highest rate of assimilation when the drug is ingested in LBFs. The food effect is identified by many parameters including physiochemical features of drug molecule, the dose, the nature of formulation, quantity and content of administered food. Post-prandial alterations in GIT that can improve drug assimilation, relative to the fasting condition, such as: (i) improved drug solubilization by BS mixed micelles and (ii) improved permeability of intestinal epithelial membrane.

Food effect can result in exaggerated pharmacological actions or unexpected toxicity, clinical trials guidelines routinely need investigations contrasting drug exposure in the fed and fasting candidates [87].

Although limited investigations demonstrate the efficacy of LBFs for justifying the food effect. Grove *et al.,* examined the food effect of seocalcitol in minipigs after ingestion of formulation either as solution in MCT, MC-SMEDDS or PG solution. Its bioavailability in the fasting state was 15%, 21% and 28% for PG, MCT and MC-SMEDDS preparations, respectively. In postprandial condition, its bioavailability from PG solution was about twice to 29% but was unchanged in comparison to the fasted condition, for both MCT and MC-SMEDDS preparations. These outcomes propose a common mechanism by which food and LBFs enhance the assimilation of PWS drugs. Other PWS drugs for which LBFs have diminished food effect on the assimilation include cyclosporine, danazol, halofantrine, DPC961, L-683, 453 *etc.* [88].

Reduction of Food Effect

Food impact can be depicted as an increment or reduction in the rate and degree of drug retention in the occurrence of food. The food impact is gaining more attention and it depends upon various components. Different perspectives, for example, improved solubility within the existence of fat parts of food, stimulation of bile discharge, surfactant impacts by food segments, delaying gastric emptying to improve the assimilation time and restraint of efflux transporters by food segments are perceived as potential instruments for bioavailability improvement of poorly soluble drugs within the presence of food. The lipid parts present in the food can provide an indistinguishable capacity as lipid segments present in the LBFs. The dietary lipids occuring in food can play a role as solubilizers for drug and consequently experience lipid digestion by gastric and pancreatic lipases that helps in the creation of different micellar species. It has been demonstrated that a couple of lipidic parts in the food can upgrade chylomicron creation and can stimulate lymphatic transport to improve bioavailability. Therefore, it is clear that if suitable lipids and surfactants are selected for the formulation of an ineffectively water-soluble drug, they can as act as substitutes for food components and consequently contesting the food impact and growing patient consistency by maintaining a strategic distance from the high-fat supper usage with dosage form. The diminishing food impact for itraconazole loaded SMEDDS was represented in 80 healthy volunteers. SMEDDS showed improved Cmax and AUC regards in both fasted and fed states when contrasted with conventional formulation of the capsule and exhibited comparable Cmax under both states showing no food impact. Also, the lessened food impact for the exceptionally lipophilic compound torcetrapib after administration in LBFs was shown. The optimized preparations indicated improved fasting condition and decreased food impact from 5-overlay to 3-overlap in dogs at dose levels of 90 mg. The optimized preparations demonstrated diminished inter-individual pharmacokinetic fluctuation [89].

Biopharmaceutical Issues

It is vital to take updates of that lipid to impact the oral bioavailability of drugs by modifying biopharmaceutical issues such as rate of disintegration and solubility in the intestinal fluids, shielding the drug from chemical and enzymatic degradation in the oil globules and development of LPs supporting lymphatic transportation of highly hydrophobic drugs.

The retention profile and the blood/lymph appropriation of the drug rely upon the number of carbons of the TG, immersion degree and the amount of the lipid ingested. Drugs retained by the intestinal lymph are typically transported to fundamental flow in relationship with the lipidic core of LPs. Despite the incitement of lymphatic transportation, the ingestion of hydrophobic drugs with lipids may improve drug assimilation into the systemetic circulation.

Specificity

In some cases, particular pharmaceutical components concentration prompts effective SESs. The viability of drug addition into a SEDDS relies upon the specific physicochemical similarity of the drug/systems. Along these lines, pre-formulation solubility and phase diagram examination are vital to get optimal formulation design [90].

CONSENT FOR PUBLICATION

Not applicable.

CONFLICT OF INTEREST

The author declares no conflict of interest, financial or otherwise.

ACKNOWLEDGEMENTS

Declared none.

REFERENCES

[1]   Miteva DO, Rutkowski JM, Dixon JB, Kilarski W, Shields JD, Swartz MA. Transmural flow modulates cell and fluid transport functions of lymphatic endothelium. Circ Res 2010; 106(5): 920-31.
        [http://dx.doi.org/10.1161/CIRCRESAHA.109.207274] [PMID: 20133901]

[2]   Iqbal J, Hussain MM. Intestinal lipid absorption. Am J Physiol Endocrinol Metab 2009; 296(6): E1183-94.
        [http://dx.doi.org/10.1152/ajpendo.90899.2008] [PMID: 19158321]

[3]   O'Driscol CM. Anatomy and physiology of the lymphatics.Lymphatic transport of medicaments. Boca Raton, FL: CRC Press Inc 1992.

[4]   Muranishi S, Fujita T, Murakami M, Yamamoto A. Potential for lymphatic targeting of peptides. J Control Release 1997; 46: 157-64.
        [http://dx.doi.org/10.1016/S0168-3659(96)01588-X]

[5]   Reddy LHV, Murthy RSR. Lymphatic transport of orally administered drugs. Indian J Exp Biol 2002; 40(10): 1097-109.
        [PMID: 12693689]

[6]   Porter CJH, Charman WN. Uptake of medicaments into the intestinal lymphatics after oral administration. Adv Drug Deliv Rev 1997; 25: 71-89.
        [http://dx.doi.org/10.1016/S0169-409X(96)00492-9]

[7]   Eldridge JH, Hammond CJ, Meulbroeck JA, Staas JK, Gilley RM, Tice TR. Controlled vaccine release in the gut-associated lymphoid tissue. I. Orally administered biodegradable microspheres target the Peyer's patches. J Control Release 1990; 11: 205-14.
        [http://dx.doi.org/10.1016/0168-3659(90)90133-E]

[8]   Hawley AE, Davis SS, Illum L. Targeting of colloids to lymph nodes: influence of lymphatic physiology and colloidal characteristics. Adv Drug Deliv Rev 1995; 17: 129-48.
        [http://dx.doi.org/10.1016/0169-409X(95)00045-9]

[9]   Beier R, Gebert A. Kinetics of particle uptake in the domes of Peyer's patches. Am J Physiol 1998; 275(1): G130-7.
        [PMID: 9655693]

[10]   Wells JM, Mercenier A. Mucosal delivery of therapeutic and prophylactic molecules using lactic acid bacteria. Nat Rev Microbiol 2008; 6(5): 349-62.
        [http://dx.doi.org/10.1038/nrmicro1840] [PMID: 18345021]

[11]   Yáñez JA, Wang SW, Knemeyer IW, Wirth MA, Alton KB. Intestinal lymphatic transport for drug delivery. Adv Drug Deliv Rev 2011; 63(10-11): 923-42.
        [http://dx.doi.org/10.1016/j.addr.2011.05.019] [PMID: 21689702]

[12]   Myers RA, Stella VJ. Factors affecting the lymphatic transport of penclomedine (NSC-338720), a lipophilic cytotoxic medicament: Comparison to DDT and hexachlorobenzene. Int J Pharm 1992; 80: 51-62.
        [http://dx.doi.org/10.1016/0378-5173(92)90261-Y]

[13]   Hauss DJ, Fogal SE, Ficorilli JV, *et al.* Lipid-based delivery systems for improving the bioavailability and lymphatic transport of a poorly water-soluble LTB4 inhibitor. J Pharm Sci 1998; 87(2): 164-9.
        [http://dx.doi.org/10.1021/js970300n] [PMID: 9519148]

[14]   Wu H, Zhou A, Lu C, Wang L. Examination of lymphatic transport of puerarin in unconscious lymph duct-cannulated rats after administration in microemulsion drug delivery systems. Eur J Pharm Sci 2011; 42(4): 348-53.
        [http://dx.doi.org/10.1016/j.ejps.2010.12.010] [PMID: 21216284]

[15]   Thakkar H, Nangesh J, Parmar M, Patel D. Formulation and characterization of lipid-based medicament delivery system of raloxifene-microemulsion and self-microemulsifying medicament delivery system. J Pharm Bioallied Sci 2011; 3: 442-8.

[http://dx.doi.org/10.4103/0975-7406.84463] [PMID: 21966167]

[16]   Takada K, Yoshimura H, Shibata N, *et al.* Effect of administration route on the selective lymphatic delivery of cyclosporin A by lipid-surfactant mixed micelles. J Pharmacobiodyn 1986; 9(2): 156-60.
[http://dx.doi.org/10.1248/bpb1978.9.156] [PMID: 3712214]

[17]   Kommuru TR, Gurley B, Khan MA, Reddy IK. Self-emulsifying drug delivery systems (SEDDS) of coenzyme Q10: formulation development and bioavailability assessment. Int J Pharm 2001; 212(2): 233-46.
[http://dx.doi.org/10.1016/S0378-5173(00)00614-1] [PMID: 11165081]

[18]   Holm R, Porter CJ, Edwards GA, Müllertz A, Kristensen HG, Charman WN. Examination of oral absorption and lymphatic transport of halofantrine in a triple-cannulated canine model after administration in self-microemulsifying drug delivery systems (SMEDDS) containing structured triglycerides. Eur J Pharm Sci 2003; 20(1): 91-7.
[http://dx.doi.org/10.1016/S0928-0987(03)00174-X] [PMID: 13678797]

[19]   Yao J, Lu Y, Zhou JP. Preparation of nobiletin in self-microemulsifying systems and its intestinal permeability in rats. J Pharm Pharm Sci 2008; 11(3): 22-9.
[http://dx.doi.org/10.18433/J3MS3M] [PMID: 18801304]

[20]   Dixit AR, Rajput SJ, Patel SG. Preparation and bioavailability assessment of SMEDDS containing valsartan. AAPS PharmSciTech 2010; 11(1): 314-21.
[http://dx.doi.org/10.1208/s12249-010-9385-0] [PMID: 20182825]

[21]   Chen Y, Li G, Wu X, *et al.* Self-microemulsifying drug delivery system (SMEDDS) of vinpocetine: formulation development and *in vivo* assessment. Biol Pharm Bull 2008; 31(1): 118-25.
[http://dx.doi.org/10.1248/bpb.31.118] [PMID: 18175953]

[22]   Li X, Yuan Q, Huang Y, Zhou Y, Liu Y. Development of silymarin self-microemulsifying drug delivery system with enhanced oral bioavailability. AAPS PharmSciTech 2010; 11(2): 672-8.
[http://dx.doi.org/10.1208/s12249-010-9432-x] [PMID: 20405254]

[23]   Sun M, Zhai X, Xue K, *et al.* Intestinal absorption and intestinal lymphatic transport of sirolimus from self-microemulsifying drug delivery systems assessed using the single-pass intestinal perfusion (SPIP) technique and a chylomicron flow blocking approach: linear correlation with oral bioavailabilities in rats. Eur J Pharm Sci 2011; 43(3): 132-40.
[http://dx.doi.org/10.1016/j.ejps.2011.04.011] [PMID: 21530655]

[24]   Singh B, Khurana L, Bandyopadhyay S, Kapil R, Katare OO. Development of optimized self-nan-
-emulsifying drug delivery systems (SNEDDS) of carvedilol with enhanced bioavailability potential. Drug Deliv 2011; 18(8): 599-612.
[http://dx.doi.org/10.3109/10717544.2011.604686] [PMID: 22008038]

[25]   Beg S, Swain S, Singh HP, Patra ChN, Rao ME. Development, optimization, and characterization of solid self-nanoemulsifying drug delivery systems of valsartan using porous carriers. AAPS PharmSciTech 2012; 13(4): 1416-27.
[http://dx.doi.org/10.1208/s12249-012-9865-5] [PMID: 23070560]

[26]   Holm R, Tønsberg H, Jørgensen EB, Abedinpour P, Farsad S, Müllertz A. Influence of bile on the absorption of halofantrine from lipid-based formulations. Eur J Pharm Biopharm 2012; 81(2): 281-7.
[http://dx.doi.org/10.1016/j.ejpb.2012.03.005] [PMID: 22465095]

[27]   Moghimi SM, Moghimi M. Enhanced lymph node retention of subcutaneously injected IgG1-PEG2000-liposomes through pentameric IgM antibody-mediated vesicular aggregation. Biochim Biophys Acta 2008; 1778(1): 51-5.
[http://dx.doi.org/10.1016/j.bbamem.2007.08.033] [PMID: 17936719]

[28]   Ling R, Li Y, Yao Q, *et al.* Lymphatic chemotherapy induces apoptosis in lymph node metastases in a rabbit breast carcinoma model. J Drug Target 2005; 13(2): 137-42.
[http://dx.doi.org/10.1080/10611860400027725] [PMID: 15823965]

[29]   Frenkel V, Etherington A, Greene M, *et al.* Delivery of liposomal doxorubicin (Doxil) in a breast cancer tumor model: investigation of potential enhancement by pulsed-high intensity focused ultrasound exposure. Acad Radiol 2006; 13(4): 469-79.
[http://dx.doi.org/10.1016/j.acra.2005.08.024] [PMID: 16554227]

[30]   O'Brien ME, Wigler N, Inbar M, *et al.* Reduced cardiotoxicity and comparable efficacy in a phase III trial of pegylated liposomal doxorubicin HCl (CAELYX/Doxil) *versus* conventional doxorubicin for first-line treatment of metastatic breast cancer. Ann Oncol 2004; 15(3): 440-9.
[http://dx.doi.org/10.1093/annonc/mdh097] [PMID: 14998846]

[31]   Ling SS, Magosso E, Khan NA, Yuen KH, Barker SA. Enhanced oral bioavailability and intestinal lymphatic transport of a hydrophilic drug using liposomes. Drug Dev Ind Pharm 2006; 32(3): 335-45.
[http://dx.doi.org/10.1080/03639040500519102] [PMID: 16556538]

[32]   Lawson KA, Anderson K, Snyder RM, *et al.* Novel vitamin E analogue and 9-nitro-camptothecin administered as liposome aerosols decrease syngeneic mouse mammary tumor burden and inhibit metastasis. Cancer Chemother Pharmacol 2004; 54(5): 421-31.
[http://dx.doi.org/10.1007/s00280-004-0817-y] [PMID: 15197487]

[33]   Latimer P, Menchaca M, Snyder RM, *et al.* Aerosol delivery of liposomal formulated paclitaxel and vitamin E analog reduces murine mammary tumor burden and metastases. Exp Biol Med (Maywood) 2009; 234(10): 1244-52.
[http://dx.doi.org/10.3181/0901-RM-8] [PMID: 19657067]

[34]   Kojima N, Biao L, Nakayama T, Ishii M, Ikehara Y, Tsujimura K. Oligomannose-coated liposomes as a therapeutic antigen-delivery and an adjuvant vehicle for induction of *in vivo* tumor immunity. J Control Release 2008; 129(1): 26-32.
[http://dx.doi.org/10.1016/j.jconrel.2008.03.023] [PMID: 18485512]

[35]   Harivardhan Reddy L, Sharma RK, Chuttani K, Mishra AK, Murthy RS. Influence of administration route on tumor uptake and biodistribution of etoposide loaded solid lipid nanoparticles in Dalton's lymphoma tumor bearing mice. J Control Release 2005; 105(3): 185-98.
[http://dx.doi.org/10.1016/j.jconrel.2005.02.028] [PMID: 15921775]

[36]   Paliwal R, Rai S, Vaidya B, *et al.* Effect of lipid core material on characteristics of solid lipid nanoparticles designed for oral lymphatic delivery. Nanomedicine (Lond) 2009; 5(2): 184-91.
[http://dx.doi.org/10.1016/j.nano.2008.08.003] [PMID: 19095502]

[37]   Zara GP, Bargoni A, Cavalli R, Fundarò A, Vighetto D, Gasco MR. Pharmacokinetics and tissue distribution of idarubicin-loaded solid lipid nanoparticles after duodenal administration to rats. J Pharm Sci 2002; 91(5): 1324-33.
[http://dx.doi.org/10.1002/jps.10129] [PMID: 11977108]

[38]   Cavalli R, Zara GP, Caputo O, Bargoni A, Fundarò A, Gasco MR. Transmucosal transport of tobramycin incorporated in SLN after duodenal administration to rats. Part I--a pharmacokinetic study. Pharmacol Res 2000; 42(6): 541-5.
[http://dx.doi.org/10.1006/phrs.2000.0737] [PMID: 11058406]

[39]   Cavalli R, Bargoni A, Podio V, Muntoni E, Zara GP, Gasco MR. Duodenal administration of solid lipid nanoparticles loaded with different percentages of tobramycin. J Pharm Sci 2003; 92(5): 1085-94.
[http://dx.doi.org/10.1002/jps.10368] [PMID: 12712429]

[40]   Chalikwar SS, Belgamwar VS, Talele VR, Surana SJ, Patil MU. Formulation and evaluation of Nimodipine-loaded solid lipid nanoparticles delivered *via* lymphatic transport system. Colloids Surf B Biointerfaces 2012; 97: 109-16.
[http://dx.doi.org/10.1016/j.colsurfb.2012.04.027] [PMID: 22609590]

[41]   Muchow M, Maincent P, Müller RH, Keck CM. Production and characterization of testosterone undecanoate-loaded NLC for oral bioavailability enhancement. Drug Dev Ind Pharm 2011; 37(1): 8-14.
[http://dx.doi.org/10.3109/03639045.2010.489559] [PMID: 21138344]

[42]   Zhuang CY, Li N, Wang M, *et al.* Preparation and characterization of vinpocetine loaded nanostructured lipid carriers (NLC) for improved oral bioavailability. Int J Pharm 2010; 394(1-2): 179-85.
[http://dx.doi.org/10.1016/j.ijpharm.2010.05.005] [PMID: 20471464]

[43]   Zhou L, Chen Y, Zhang Z, He J, Du M, Wu Q. Preparation of tripterine nanostructured lipid carriers and their absorption in rat intestine. Pharmazie 2012; 67(4): 304-10.
[PMID: 22570936]

[44]   Kim H, Kim Y, Lee J. Liposomal formulations for enhanced lymphatic medicament delivery. Eur J Pharm Sci 2013; 8(2): 96-03.

[45]   Ali Khan A, Mudassir J, Mohtar N, Darwis Y. Advanced drug delivery to the lymphatic system: lipid-based nanoformulations. Int J Nanomedicine 2013; 8: 2733-44.
[PMID: 23926431]

[46]   Hawley AE, Illum L, Davis SS. The effect of lymphatic oedema on the uptake of colloids to the lymph nodes. Biopharm Drug Dispos 1998; 19(3): 193-7.
[http://dx.doi.org/10.1002/(SICI)1099-081X(199804)19:3<193::AID-BDD88>3.0.CO;2-V] [PMID: 9570003]

[47]   Luo G, Yu X, Jin C, *et al.* LyP-1-conjugated nanoparticles for targeting drug delivery to lymphatic metastatic tumors. Int J Pharm 2010; 385(1-2): 150-6.
[http://dx.doi.org/10.1016/j.ijpharm.2009.10.014] [PMID: 19825404]

[48]   Oussoren C, Zuidema J, Crommelin DJ, Storm G. Lymphatic uptake and biodistribution of liposomes after subcutaneous injection. II. Influence of liposomal size, lipid compostion and lipid dose. Biochim Biophys Acta 1997; 1328(2): 261-72.
[http://dx.doi.org/10.1016/S0005-2736(97)00122-3] [PMID: 9315622]

[49]   Takakura Y, Hashida M, Sezaki H. Anatomy and physiology of the lymphatics.Lymphatic transport of drug. Boca Raton, FL: CRC Press Inc 1992.

[50]   Kaminskas LM, Porter CJ. Targeting the lymphatics using dendritic polymers (dendrimers). Adv Drug Deliv Rev 2011; 63(10-11): 890-900.
[http://dx.doi.org/10.1016/j.addr.2011.05.016] [PMID: 21683746]

[51]   Clogston JD, Patri AK. Zeta potential measurement. Methods Mol Biol 2011; 697: 63-70.
[http://dx.doi.org/10.1007/978-1-60327-198-1_6] [PMID: 21116954]

[52]   Kaur CD, Nahar M, Jain NK. Lymphatic targeting of zidovudine using surface-engineered liposomes. J Drug Target 2008; 16(10): 798-805.
[http://dx.doi.org/10.1080/10611860802475688] [PMID: 19005941]

[53]   Patel HM, Boodle KM, Vaughan-Jones R. Assessment of the potential uses of liposomes for lymphoscintigraphy and lymphatic drug delivery. Failure of 99m-technetium marker to represent intact liposomes in lymph nodes. Biochim Biophys Acta 1984; 801(1): 76-86.
[http://dx.doi.org/10.1016/0304-4165(84)90214-9] [PMID: 6087919]

[54]   Hawley AE, Illum L, Davis SS. Preparation of biodegradable, surface engineered PLGA nanospheres with enhanced lymphatic drainage and lymph node uptake. Pharm Res 1997; 14(5): 657-61.
[http://dx.doi.org/10.1023/A:1012117531448] [PMID: 9165539]

[55]   Dahlbäck B, Hermansson M, Kjelleberg S, Norkrans B. The hydrophobicity of bacteria - an important factor in their initial adhesion at the air-water interface. Arch Microbiol 1981; 128(3): 267-70.
[http://dx.doi.org/10.1007/BF00422527] [PMID: 7212931]

[56]   Charman WN, Stella VJ. Estimating the maximum potential for intestinal lymphatic transport of lipophilic medicament molecules. Int J Pharm 1986; 34: 175-8.
[http://dx.doi.org/10.1016/0378-5173(86)90027-X]

[57]   Ruckmani K, Sivakumar M, Ganeshkumar PA. Methotrexate loaded solid lipid nanoparticles (SLN)

for effective treatment of carcinoma. J Nanosci Nanotechnol 2006; 6(9-10): 2991-5.
[http://dx.doi.org/10.1166/jnn.2006.457] [PMID: 17048509]

[58] Sanjula B, Shah FM, Javed A, Alka A. Effect of poloxamer 188 on lymphatic uptake of carvedilol-loaded solid lipid nanoparticles for bioavailability enhancement. J Drug Target 2009; 17(3): 249-56.
[http://dx.doi.org/10.1080/10611860902718672] [PMID: 19255893]

[59] Boyd M, Risovic V, Jull P, Choo E, Wasan KM. A stepwise surgical procedure to investigate the lymphatic transport of lipid-based oral drug formulations: Cannulation of the mesenteric and thoracic lymph ducts within the rat. J Pharmacol Toxicol Methods 2004; 49(2): 115-20.
[http://dx.doi.org/10.1016/j.vascn.2003.11.004] [PMID: 14990336]

[60] Dahmani FZ, Yang H, Zhou J, Yao J, Zhang T, Zhang Q. Enhanced oral bioavailability of paclitaxel in pluronic/LHR mixed polymeric micelles: preparation, *in vitro* and *in vivo* evaluation. Eur J Pharm Sci 2012; 47(1): 179-89.
[http://dx.doi.org/10.1016/j.ejps.2012.05.015] [PMID: 22683386]

[61] Dahan A, Hoffman A. Rationalizing the selection of oral lipid based drug delivery systems by an *in vitro* dynamic lipolysis model for improved oral bioavailability of poorly water soluble drugs. J Control Release 2008; 129(1): 1-10.
[http://dx.doi.org/10.1016/j.jconrel.2008.03.021] [PMID: 18499294]

[62] Trevaskis NL, Charman WN, Porter CJ. Lipid-based delivery systems and intestinal lymphatic drug transport: a mechanistic update. Adv Drug Deliv Rev 2008; 60(6): 702-16.
[http://dx.doi.org/10.1016/j.addr.2007.09.007] [PMID: 18155316]

[63] Yáñez JA, Wang SW, Knemeyer IW, Wirth MA, Alton KB. Intestinal lymphatic transport for drug delivery. Adv Drug Deliv Rev 2011; 63(10-11): 923-42.
[http://dx.doi.org/10.1016/j.addr.2011.05.019] [PMID: 21689702]

[64] O'Driscoll CM. Lipid-based formulations for intestinal lymphatic delivery. Eur J Pharm Sci 2002; 15(5): 405-15.
[http://dx.doi.org/10.1016/S0928-0987(02)00051-9] [PMID: 12036717]

[65] Seeballuck F, Ashford MB, O'Driscoll CM. The effects of pluronics block copolymers and Cremophor EL on intestinal lipoprotein processing and the potential link with P-glycoprotein in Caco-2 cells. Pharm Res 2003; 20(7): 1085-92.
[http://dx.doi.org/10.1023/A:1024422625596] [PMID: 12880295]

[66] Seeballuck F, Lawless E, Ashford MB, O'Driscoll CM. Stimulation of triglyceride-rich lipoprotein secretion by polysorbate 80: *in vitro* and *in vivo* correlation using Caco-2 cells and a cannulated rat intestinal lymphatic model. Pharm Res 2004; 21(12): 2320-6.
[http://dx.doi.org/10.1007/s11095-004-7684-4] [PMID: 15648264]

[67] Karpf DM, Holm R, Garafalo C, Levy E, Jacobsen J, Müllertz A. Effect of different surfactants in biorelevant medium on the secretion of a lipophilic compound in lipoproteins using Caco-2 cell culture. J Pharm Sci 2006; 95(1): 45-55.
[http://dx.doi.org/10.1002/jps.20431] [PMID: 16307455]

[68] Gershkovich P, Hoffman A. Uptake of lipophilic drugs by plasma derived isolated chylomicrons: linear correlation with intestinal lymphatic bioavailability. Eur J Pharm Sci 2005; 26(5): 394-404.
[http://dx.doi.org/10.1016/j.ejps.2005.07.011] [PMID: 16140514]

[69] Holm R, Hoest J. Successful in silico predicting of intestinal lymphatic transfer. Int J Pharm 2004; 272(1-2): 189-93.
[http://dx.doi.org/10.1016/j.ijpharm.2003.12.017] [PMID: 15019082]

[70] Edwards GA, Porter CJH, Caliph SM, Khoo SM, Charman WN. Animal models for the study of intestinal lymphatic drug transport. Adv Drug Deliv Rev 2001; 50(1-2): 45-60.
[http://dx.doi.org/10.1016/S0169-409X(01)00148-X] [PMID: 11489333]

[71] Brocks DR, Davies NM. Lymphatic drug absorption *via* the enterocytes: Pharmacokinetic simulation,

modeling, and considerations for optimal drug development. J Pharm Pharm Sci 2018; 21(1s): 254s-70s.
[http://dx.doi.org/10.18433/jpps30217] [PMID: 30348249]

[72]   Dahan A, Hoffman A. Evaluation of a chylomicron flow blocking approach to investigate the intestinal lymphatic transport of lipophilic drugs. Eur J Pharm Sci 2005; 24(4): 381-8.
[http://dx.doi.org/10.1016/j.ejps.2004.12.006] [PMID: 15734305]

[73]   Cai S, Xie Y, Bagby TR, Cohen MS, Forrest ML. Intralymphatic chemotherapy using a hyaluronan-cisplatin conjugate. J Surg Res 2008; 147(2): 247-52.
[http://dx.doi.org/10.1016/j.jss.2008.02.048] [PMID: 18498877]

[74]   Dokania S, Joshi AK. Self-microemulsifying drug delivery system (SMEDDS)--challenges and road ahead. Drug Deliv 2015; 22(6): 675-90.
[http://dx.doi.org/10.3109/10717544.2014.896058] [PMID: 24670091]

[75]   Verma R, Kaushik D. *In vitro* lipolysis as a tool for establishment of IVIVC for lipid based drug delivery systems. Curr Drug Deliv 2019; 16(8): 688-97.
[http://dx.doi.org/10.2174/1567201816666190620115716] [PMID: 31250755]

[76]   Hörter D, Dressman JB. Influence of physicochemical properties on dissolution of drugs in the gastrointestinal tract. Adv Drug Deliv Rev 2001; 46(1-3): 75-87.
[PMID: 11259834]

[77]   Siepmann J, Siepmann F. Mathematical modeling of drug dissolution. Int J Pharm 2013; 453(1): 12-24.
[http://dx.doi.org/10.1016/j.ijpharm.2013.04.044] [PMID: 23618956]

[78]   Dressman JB, Reppas C. *In vitro-in vivo* correlations for lipophilic, poorly water-soluble drugs. Eur J Pharm Sci 2000; 11 (Suppl. 2): S73-80.
[http://dx.doi.org/10.1016/S0928-0987(00)00181-0] [PMID: 11033429]

[79]   Alexander JS, Ganta VC, Jordan PA, Witte MH. Gastrointestinal lymphatics in health and disease. Pathophysiology 2010; 17(4): 315-35.
[http://dx.doi.org/10.1016/j.pathophys.2009.09.003] [PMID: 20022228]

[80]   Barrett K, Brooks H, Boitano S, Barman S. Blood as a circulatory fluid & the dynamics of blood and lymph flow Ganong's review of medical physiology. New York: McGraw Hill 2009; pp. 550-62.

[81]   Charman WN, Noguchi T, Stella VJ. An experimental system designed to study the in situ intestinal lymphatic transport of lipophilic medicaments in anesthetized rats. Int J Pharm 1986; 33: 155-64.
[http://dx.doi.org/10.1016/0378-5173(86)90049-9]

[82]   Oussoren C, Storm G. Liposomes to target the lymphatics by subcutaneous administration. Adv Drug Deliv Rev 2001; 50(1-2): 143-56.
[http://dx.doi.org/10.1016/S0169-409X(01)00154-5] [PMID: 11489337]

[83]   Caliph SM, Charman WN, Porter CJH. Effect of short-, medium-, and long-chain fatty acid-based vehicles on the absolute oral bioavailability and intestinal lymphatic transport of halofantrine and assessment of mass balance in lymph-cannulated and non-cannulated rats. J Pharm Sci 2000; 89(8): 1073-84.
[http://dx.doi.org/10.1002/1520-6017(200008)89:8<1073::AID-JPS12>3.0.CO;2-V]
[PMID: 10906731]

[84]   Khoo SM, Humberstone AJ, Porter CJH, *et al*. Formulation design and bioavailability assessment of lipidic self-emulsifying formulations of halofantrine. Int J Pharm 1998; 167: 155-64.
[http://dx.doi.org/10.1016/S0378-5173(98)00054-4]

[85]   Porter CJ. Drug delivery to the lymphatic system. Crit Rev Ther Drug Carrier Syst 1997; 14(4): 333-93.
[PMID: 9450175]

[86]   Ichihashi T, Kinoshita H, Yamada H. Absorption and disposition of epithiosteroids in rats (2):

Avoidance of first-pass metabolism of mepitiostane by lymphatic absorption. Xenobiotica 1991; 21(7): 873-80.
[http://dx.doi.org/10.3109/00498259109039527] [PMID: 1776263]

[87]   Hauss DJ, Ed. Oral lipid-based formulations: Enhancing the bioavailability of poorly water.
[http://dx.doi.org/10.3109/9781420017267]

[88]   Grove M, Müllertz A, Pedersen GP, Nielsen JL. Bioavailability of seocalcitol III. Administration of lipid-based formulations to minipigs in the fasted and fed state. Eur J Pharm Sci 2007; 31(1): 8-15.
[http://dx.doi.org/10.1016/j.ejps.2007.01.007] [PMID: 17383165]

[89]   Porter CJ, Charman WN. Intestinal lymphatic drug transport: an update. Adv Drug Deliv Rev 2001; 50(1-2): 61-80.
[http://dx.doi.org/10.1016/S0169-409X(01)00151-X] [PMID: 11489334]

[90]   Tang B, Cheng G, Gu JC, Xu CH. Development of solid self-emulsifying drug delivery systems: preparation techniques and dosage forms. Drug Discov Today 2008; 13(13-14): 606-12.
[http://dx.doi.org/10.1016/j.drudis.2008.04.006] [PMID: 18598917]

CHAPTER 6

Advantages, Marketed Formulations and Evaluation Parameters of SMEDDS

Deepak Kaushik[1,*], Ravinder Verma[1], Vineet Mittal[1] and Deepika Purohit[2]

[1] *Department of Pharmaceutical Sciences, Maharshi Dayanand University, Rohtak (Haryana), 124001, India*

[2] *Department of Pharmaceutical Sciences, Indra Gandhi University, Meerpur, Rewari, India*

Abstract: Various applications of SMEDDS are discussed in detail in this chapter, which include: upgrading the solubility and bioavailability, protection against biodegradation, effortless production and scale-up, diminishment in inter-subject and intra-subject inconstancy and food impacts, the capability to convey peptides that are liable to enzymatic hydrolysis in GIT, no impact on the lipid digestion and improvement in drug loading capability. Different variables affecting the performance of SMEDDS formulation are the nature, amount of the drug, polarity of the lipophilic phase, and a charge on a droplet of emulsion. Globule size, percent transmission, robust dilution, zeta potential measurement, cloud point estimation, stability studies, *in vitro* lipolysis, *in vitro* drug release assessment, permeability study, *etc.*, are various evaluation parameters for SMEDDS/LBDDS that are discussed briefly. This chapter highlights various advantages, evaluation parameters, and marketed products related to SMEDDS.

Keywords: Digestion of lipids, Enzymatic hydrolysis, Food effect, Globule size, *In vitro* lipolysis, Solubility equilibrium.

APPLICATIONS OF SMEDDS

There are various applications of SMEDDS, which are discussed below in detail:

Upgrading Solubility and Bioavailability

When the drug is formulated in SMEDDS, it improves solubility because it avoids the dissolution step. In SMEDDS, the matrix reacts with water to produce a fine o/w emulsion. The drug will be transported to GI mucosa by this emulsion in the dissolved form and is available for assimilation. In this manner, increment in bio-

---

[*] **Corresponding author Deepak Kaushik:** Department of Pharmaceutical Sciences, Maharshi Dayanand University, Rohtak (Haryana), 124001, India; Tel: +91 9315809626; E-mail: deepkaushik1977@gmail.com

availability is seen with numerous drugs when they are formulated as SMEDDS dosage form [1].

Protection Against Biodegradation

The potential of SMEDDS to diminish degradation and enhance retention might be particularly valuable for BCS class II and IV drugs that have less solubility, degradation in GIT, and less oral bioavailability. Numerous drugs are destroyed in the biological system as a result of an acidic environment of the stomach, hydrolytic degradation, enzymatic degradation, *etc.* When drugs are developed as SMEDDS, they can protect the degradation of drugs by forming LCP in SMEDDS that may act as a boundary between degrading milieu and the drug [2].

Ex: Acetylsalicylic acid is a drug that degrades in GIT resulting in salicylic acid production in acidic milieu after hydrolyzation. Its oral bioavailability is enhanced by 73% by Galacticles Oral Lipid Matrix.

Low Cost of Production and Ease of Scale-up

The simplicity of production and scale are some of the key features that make SMEDDS novel when compared with other DDSs like SDs, liposomes, nanoparticles, and so on. SMEDDS involve simple and economical manufacturing process such as a blender with agitator and volumetric liquid filling instrument for pilot-scale fabricating [3].

Diminishment of Inter/intra-subject Variability and Food Effects

A few drugs that indicate extensive inter-subject/intra-subject variation in retention result in diminished efficiency of drug and the patient compliance. Food is the key factor influencing the therapeutic potential of drugs in the body. SMEDDS are beneficial for these drugs. A few research works authenticated that their performance has no impact on food, and give reproducibility of plasma profile [4].

Capability to Convey Peptides that are Liable to Enzymatic Hydrolysis in GIT

One exciting feature that marks them better as compared to other DDS is their capacity to convey macromolecules such as peptides, hormones, protein substances, and inhibitors and their capacity to propose security from enzymatic hydrolysis. The intestinal hydrolysis of prodrug by cholinesterase can be secured using Tween 20, a surfactant used in microemulsion products. These systems are created without the help of energy or warming, subsequently reasonable for thermolabile drugs such as peptides and hormones [5].

No Impact of Lipid Digestion Mechanism

Dissimilar to the next LBDDS, the efficiency of SMEDDS is not affected by lipolysis, bile salts (BS) that aid in emulsification, the activity of pancreatic lipases, and the blended micelle formation. These are not assimilated before the drug as they contain the drug in microemulsion formulation, which can go through the mucin and aqueous undisturbed/unstirred layer of water [6].

Improved Drug Loading Capacity

SMEDDS provides improved drug loading capacity when compared with traditional lipid formulation as the solubility of inadequately water-soluble drugs with a partition coefficient (2<log P>4) is generally less in natural lipids and significantly more in amphiphilic ingredients [7].

Supersaturable SMEDDS (s-SMEDDS)

The presence of high surfactant concentration in these formulations can prompt GI irritation. Another class of supersaturable formulations, including s-SMEDDS, has been composed and created to diminish side-effects of surfactants and accomplish fast retention of inadequately soluble drugs. The s-SMEDDS strategy is to produce an extended supersaturated formation of the drug at the point when the preparation is discharged from a suitable dosage form into a fluid media. Supersaturation is governed to expand the thermodynamic potential of the drug that affects its solubility capacity, to bring about an expanded dynamic force to transit and cross biological barriers [8].

MECHANISM OF SELF-EMULSIFICATION

This is related to free energy that is represented by ΔG, as given in the below equation:

$$\Delta G = \Sigma \, N \, \pi \, r2 \, \sigma$$

The system, usually named SMEDDS, has not yet been appeared to emulsify immediately in the thermodynamic sense. Pouton has stated that the emulsification feature of the surfactant might be identified with the phase inversion behavior of the system. At the phase inversion temperature, the surfactant is highly mobile; thus, the o/w interfacial energy is diminished, prompting a diminishment in energy which is essential for emulsification [9].

Traditional emulsions are created by blending two immiscible liquids, essentially water and oil which are balanced out by the surfactant. At the point when an emulsion creation occurs,, surface area extension is made between two phases.

The surfactant particles will create a film around the core phase of the globule to stabilize the emulsion. In conventional emulsion, the surface free energy relies upon the size of droplets and interfacial tension during their development. If the emulsion isn't balanced out by surfactants, at that point, both phases will split as interfacial pressure and free energy of the system decreases. In the case of SMEDDS, free energy ocreation is either low or positive or even negative that brings about emulsification. Incorporation of binary mixture (oil/non-ionic surfactant) to water results in the development of an interface between both phases. It has been discovered that self-emulsification (SE) occurs due to the entrance of water into the LCP that is created at the oil/surfactant-water interface into which water can enter assisted by delicate agitation during SE. After water permeation to a specific farthest point (degree), it brings about the disruption of the interface and creates globules. This LC phase is accountable for the high stability of resultant nanoemulsion against the mixture. This phase is favorable for the high stability of these emulsions. "Reiss has recommended that SE occurs when entropy change that favors dispersion is more than the energy needed for building the surface region of the dispersion. Development of emulsion leads to free energy, which is a direct function of energy needed to make another surface between two phases [10]."

It is obvious from the equation that the unconstrained development of an interface between the oil and water phase is energetically not promising. Where ΔG is the free energy related to the process. It is obvious from the above equation that spontaneous development of the interface between the oil and water phase isn't positive because of greater energy levels. The system usually categorized as SMEDDS has not yet been appeared to emulsify suddenly in an evident thermodynamic sense [11].

Groves and Mustafa built up a technique for quantitative evaluation of simplicity of emulsification by observing turbidity of an oil-surfactant system in aqueous media, utilizing phosphate nonylphenoxylate and fatty alcohol ethoxylate in n-hexane and recommended that this procedure might be related to the ease with which water penetrates oil-water interface, due to the development of LCP at the interface, that resuls in emulsification [12].

FACTORS INFLUENCING SMEDDS

Different variables are impacting the performance of SMEDDS formulation. The quantities of the drug, polarity of the phase, the solubility of the drug and charge on droplet are the fundamental elements influencing SMEDDS, which are shown in Fig. (**1**) and discussed below:

Nature and Amount of the Drug

Drugs that are ingested at high dosage are not reasonable unless they display a great degree solubility in not less than one of their ingredients, ideally the lipophilic phase. The drugs which show less solubility in aqueous and lipid dosage (ordinarily with low log P values) are not easy to be conveyed by these systems. Their capacity to keep up the drug in the solubilized state is extraordinarily impacted by the drug solubility in the oily phase. As specified above, if surfactant/co-surfactant participates prominently in drug solubilization, there may be a threat of precipitation, as their dilution will prompt decreasing the capacity of the surfactant/co-surfactant. Equilibrium solubility estimations can be completed to expect potential instances of precipitation in the gut. Nonetheless, crystallization can be delayed in solubilizing and colloidal stabilizing milieu of GIT. Pouton says that equilibrium can be achieved up to five days in such preparations and the drug can stay in a super-saturated form for up to one day after starting the emulsification process. In this manner, it can be contended that such items are not liable to result in the precipitation of the drug in GIT before the drug is assimilated and in reality, that super-saturate can upgrade retention by expanding the thermodynamic action of the medicament. There is a requirement for applied processes to anticipate the destiny of medicaments after the scattering of lipid systems in the GIT [13].

Polarity of the Lipophilic Phase

This factor governs the drug discharge from the microemulsions, which is affected by HLB, the number of carbon atoms, level of unsaturation of unsaturated fat, the molecular weight of hydrophilic part and the concentration of emulsifier. In reality the polarity shows the affinity of a drug for oil, water and the kind of forces created. The high polarity will improve fast release rate of the drug into aqueous media. This is affirmed by the perceptions of Sang-Cheol Chi, who found that the release rate of idebenone from SMEDDS is reliant on the polarity of the oil phase utilized. The most elevated discharge rate was attained by the preparation that had the oil phase with the maximum polarity [14].

The most elevated release is achieved with the preparation that had an oily phase with the most noteworthy polarity. Equilibrium solubility estimation can be done to suspect possible instances of precipitation in GIT. Be that as it may, crystallization could be moderate in solubilizing and colloidal stabilizing out the condition of the gut [15].

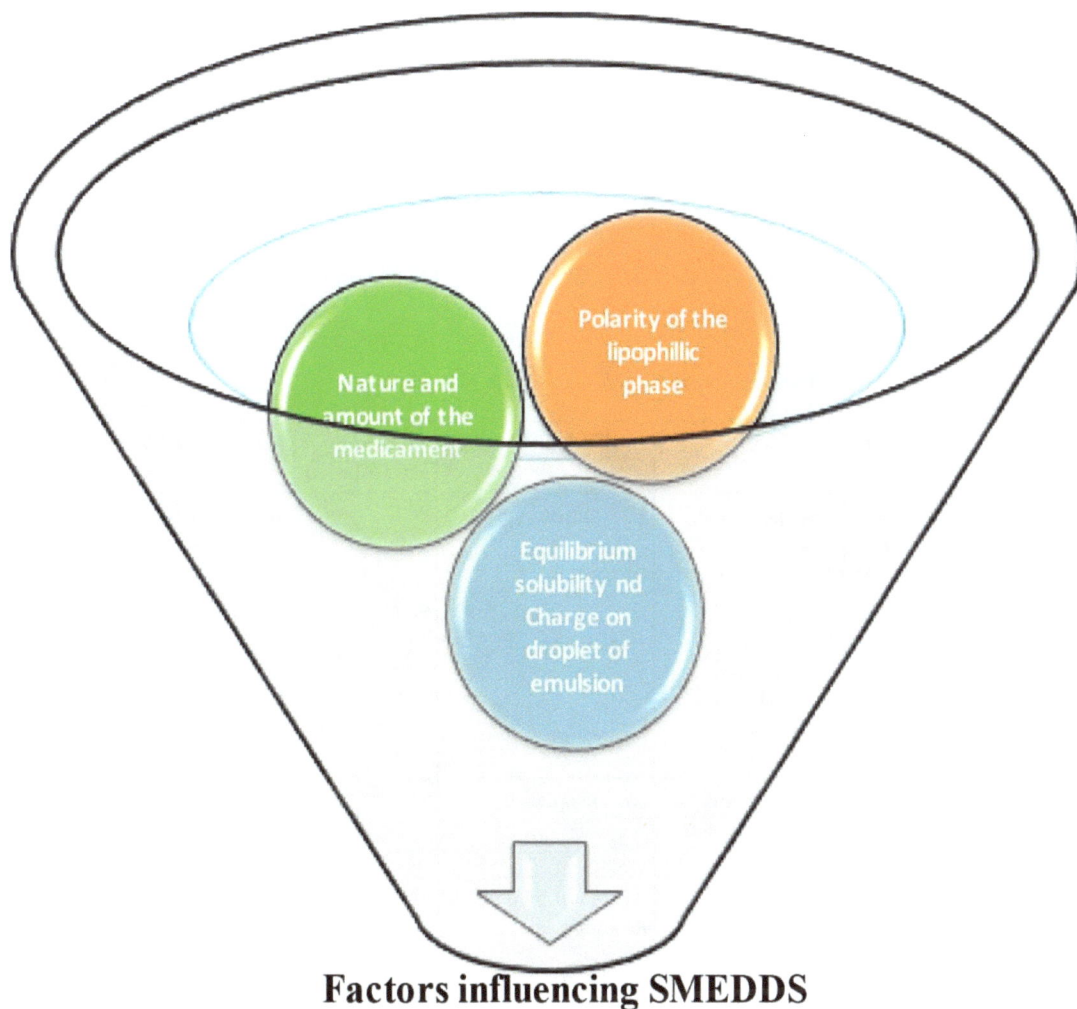

Fig. (1). Fundamental elements influencing SMEDDS.

Solubility Equailibrium

Their capacity to keep the drug in the solubilized state is enormously impacted by the drug solubility in the oil phase. If surfactant/co-surfactant is added in higher amount in drug solubilization, there can be a threat of precipitation because their dilution will prompt bringing down of dissolvable limit of the surfactant/co-surfactant. The estimate of solubility at equilibrium can be done by checking potential instances of precipitation in the GIT.

Charge on Droplet of Emulsion

Many physiological investigations demonstrated that the apical capability of absorptive cells and also all different cells in the body have a negative (-ve) charge w.r.t. a mucosal solution in lumen. The charge might be positive in a few formulations, which expands retention because of the improvement of electrostatic charge [10].

There are various marketed formulations of SMEDDS [16, 17]. Some marketed products are represented in Table **1**.

Table 1. Some marketed Pharmaceutical products based on SEDDS.

Drug	Ingredients	Indication	Type of Formulation	Tradename/Company
Saquinavir	Medium-chain povidone, mono-diglycerides, dl---tocopherol	HIV anti-viral	SGC	Fortovase (Roche)
Lopinavir and Ritonavir	Acesulfame potassium, alcohol, glycerin, Citric acid, high fructose corn syrup, peppermint oil, Cremophore RH 40, povidone, PG	HIV anti-viral	SGC	Kaletra (Abbott)
Bexarotene	Polyethylene glycol 400, polysorbate 20, povidone, BHA	Anti-neoplastic	SGC	Targretin (Ligand)
Tretinoin	Soybean oil, BHA, edetate disodium, methylparaben, propylparaben	Acute pro-myelocytic leukemia	SGC	Vesanoid (Roche)
Cyclosporine A	dl-α-tocopherol, corn oil-mono-di-triglycerides, cremophore RH 40	Immuno-suppressant	SGC	Neoral® (Novartis)
Cyclosporine A	Polyoxyl 35 castor oil (cremophor EL), polysorbate 80	Immuno-suppressant	HGC	Gengraf (Abbott)
Fenofibrate	Lauryl macrogol-glycerides	Anti-hyperlipidemic	HGC	Lipirex (Sanofi-Aventis)
Ibuprofen	Lauryl macrogol-glycerides	NSAIDs	HGC	Solufen (Sanofi-Aventis)

EVALUATION PARAMETERS

The prime means for self-micro emulsification judgment is visual assessment. The effectiveness of self-micro emulsification can be evaluated by various parameters as shown in Fig. (**2**).

Different assessment parameters evaluated in SMEDDS are the following:

Globule Size Estimation

The microemulsion globule size is estimated by photon correlation spectroscopy (PCS) or scanning electron microscopy (SEM), laser diffraction and coulter counter, which can determine the size of 10 to 5000 nm. Globule size of emulsion is an essential feature since it decides the rate and degree of drug discharge and drug assimilation. PCS or SEM is helpful equipment for assurance of emulsion droplet estimate, particularly when features of emulsion don't alter upon infinite aqueous dilution. The globule size distribution is the most imperative attribute of the *in vivo* fate of medicated emulsion [18].

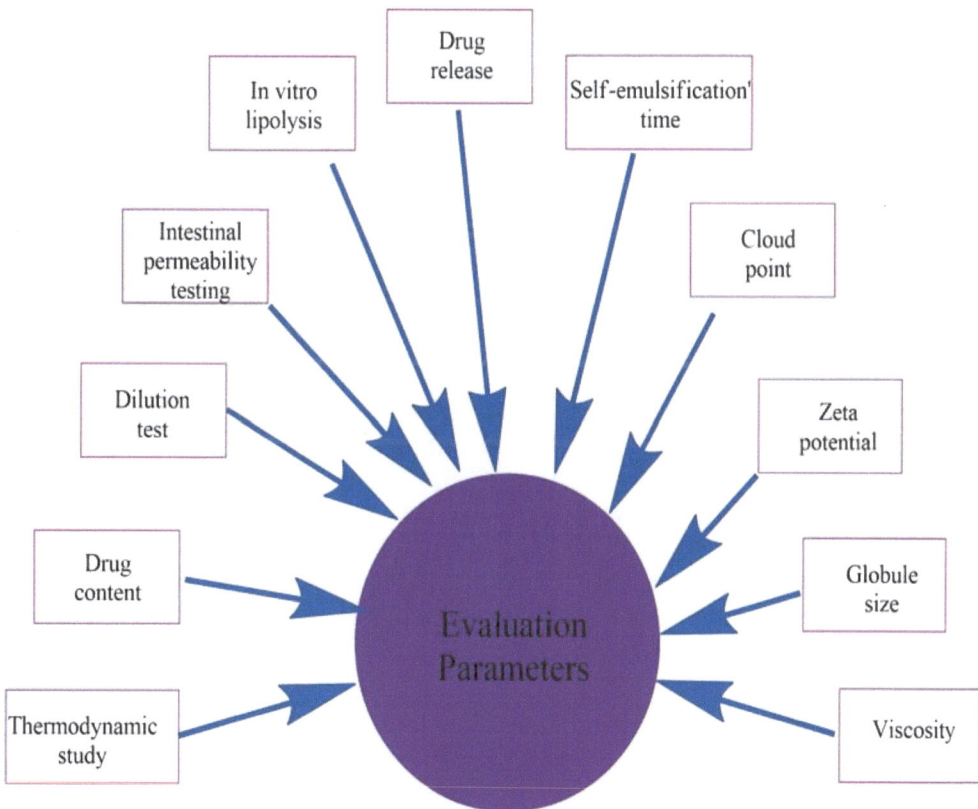

Fig. (2). Various evaluation parameters for SMEDDS.

Small-angle Neutron Scattering

It can be utilized to get data on the size and shape of the globules [19].

Refractive Index and Percent Transmission

The refractive index exhibits the clarity of the formulation. It is estimated by a refractometer. UV-Vis spectrophotometer is utilized to estimate the percentage of transmittance at a particular wavelength keeping distilled water as blank. The refractive index of formulation ought to resemble water. If formulation is demonstrating transmittance more than 99 percent, then, it is supposed to be transparent [20, 21].

Robustness Dilution

SMEDDS/SNEDDS needs to guarantee that emulsion/nanoemulsion created has comparative features at various dilutions to accomplish a constant drug discharge profile and guarantee that the drug won't get hastened at higher dilutions *in vivo* which may fundamentally impede the assimilation of the drug from preparation. SMEDDS ought to be assessed by dilution at various dilutions and exploring their impact on characteristics of produced emulsion/ nanoemulsion [22, 23].

Zeta Potential Estimation

Zeta potential is assumed an important part of bioavailability since the charge of oil droplets interacts with luminal intestinal mucosal cells as they are negatively charged, which influences retention and bioavailability because of the development of the electrostatic charge. It is measured by utilizing Zeta sizer in triplicate tests. There is a fundamentally negative charge in SMEDDS because of the occurrence of free FA. Zeta potential might be positive or negative on the foundation or basis of oil and surfactant proportion [24].

This is utilized to determine the charge of the globules. The charge of globules in SMEDDS is a feature that ought to be evaluated. For the most part, the expansion in electrostatic repulsion forces among droplets of nanoemulsion avoids the coalescence of these globules. The zeta potential of SMEDDS is normally estimated by utilizing Malvern Zeta Sizer on behalf of electrophoresis and electrical conductivity of produced nanoemulsion [25].

Zeta potential is ascertained by Helmholtz-Smoluchowski Equation 1:

$$U=\varepsilon\xi Ex/\mu$$
U = Electrophoretic speed
ε = permittivity
ξ = Zeta potential
μ = Viscosity
Ex = Axial electric field

(1)

Oil globules have a charge that is another property of SMEDDS that ought to be evaluated. The oil globules charge in customary SMEDDS is negative because of the free unsaturated fats; be that as it may, joining of a cationic lipid, for example, oleylamine will give cationic SMEDDS. Subsequently, these systems have a potential estimation of around 35-45 mV. This positive n-potential esteem is conserved after the addition of the drug candidates.

Electroconductivity Study

This test is done for the estimation of the electroconductive nature of the system. It is estimated by electro conductometer. The higher value demonstrates the o/w type of emulsion and brings lesser value demonstrates w/o type of emulsion. In SMEDDS, oil globules contain negative charges due to the occurrence of free unsaturated fats [26].

Turbidimetric Assessment

It is a factor for the assurance of droplet size and self-emulsification time. Turbidimetric assessment is carried out to examine the development of droplets after emulsification. The predetermined quantity of SMEDDS is incorporated into a predetermined amount of appropriate medium under ceaseless mixing on a magnetic stirrer at 50 rpm at optimum temperature and a turbidimeter is used for assessment of turbidity.

Effect of Dilution at various pH

This investigation is performed at various pH such as 1.2, 7.4 and 12 to get the effect of dilution on SMEDDS preconcentrate, with a particular objective to relevant physiological dilution strategy later than oral ingestion. In this, dilution is done (10 and 100 times) and visual recognition is recorded [16, 27].

Impact of Temperature

The self-emulsification process appears to be particular to the temperature at which self-emulsification comes about. Hence, the impact of temperature on the droplet size can likewise be researched [28].

Determination of Viscosity

The rheological features (viscosity, flow and thixotropy) of the formulation are measured by rotational viscometers, digital instruments such as cup and bob, or coaxial viscosity apparatus for the determination of viscosity. These are utilized for assurance of viscosity of fresh and different SMEDDS formulations, which have been put away for a longer period.

Oscillating, Brookfield viscometer can be utilized for measuring this parameter. SMEDDS are filled in SGC/HGC [29].

The viscosity measurement assures whether the system is o/w or w/o. The system is less viscous, then it is o/w type of the system and assuming high viscous, then it is w/o system. These can be filled in SGC, where, it ought to have significant flow features for flowing.

Hard or soft gelatin capsules are utilized for filling the liquid SMEDDS that evaluate its filling capacity in them. If the system has less viscosity, it might improve the possibility of escaping from the capsule and a system with high viscosity may cause difficulty in pourability [30].

Cloud Point Estimation

It is an essential feature in SMEDDS comprising of non-ionic surfactants. When the temperature is greater than the cloud point, a permanent phase partition will happen and the shiftiness of the arrangement would severely affect the drug ingestion due to the drying out of its concentrations. Consequently, the cloud point for these formulations ought to be over 37°C, which will maintain a strategic distance from phase partition, happening in the gastrointestinal tract [31].

Cloud point occurs because of the dehydration of polyoxyethylene oxide part of non–ionic surfactant. It is a vital feature in SMEDDS comprising of non-ionic surfactants when the temperature is greater than the cloud point, 0.5 ml of pre-concentrate is diluted to 50 ml with distilled water in a glass receptacle and warms at the rate of 0.5°C/min in a water bath, and temperature at which dispersion turns cloudy is considered as Tc. After the temperature surpasses the cloud point, cool the sample underneath Tc and afterward warm it again to ensure the reproducibility of outcomes [12].

Centrifugation Stability Evaluation

This evaluation can be utilized to decide the strength of SMEDDS after emulsion development. Samples are diluted with purified water, which is further centrifuged at fixed rpm for a determined time and after that analyzed for the phase partitioning [32].

Dye Solubilization Test

The portrayal of SMEDDS can be evaluated using dye solubilization. This evaluation is utilized to distinguish the type of developed nanoemulsion and its continuous phase. For this, the water-soluble dye is spread onto the surface of the formed nanoemulsion. By watching the scattering of dye or the cluster development, the nature of the internal and external phase of emulsion can be found [33].

TEM Analysis

The morphology of the nanoemulsion acquired from SMEDDS is explored utilizing this instrument [31].

Dispersibility Test

The effectiveness of the self-emulsification of the formulation is estimated employing a USP dissolution apparatus. After dilution, 500 times of the preparation with water is to be incorporated at 37±0.5°C in USP II pivoting at 50 rpm with moderate agitation. *In vitro* performance of formulation is assessed from such a scattering utilizing a reasonable grading system. The grading system can be found on the arrangement of a microemulsion (o/w or w/o), micro-emulsion gel, emulsion or emulgel [1, 12].

Impact of Drug Loading on Droplet Size

Microemulsion is developed utilizing the optimized composition of the formulation, formulated with or without drug for the estimation of this parameter. The resultant 0.5 ml SMEDDS preconcentrate is diluted up to 100 ml with double distilled water and the average droplet size of the consequent microemulsion is measured *via* Zeta sizer [34].

Drug Content Estimation

The drug is extracted from pre-measured SMEDDS by dissolving in an appropriate solvent. At that point, the solvent extract is investigated for drug substances by reasonable diagnostic techniques against the standard solvent solution of the drug [19].

In Vitro Lipolysis

This examination is conducted to expose formulation in the digestive tract under a state of fed or fasting condition, to get the drug solubilization and drug discharge in the intestine. It is conducted by employing as a part of the *in vitro* lipid digestion model with a pH-Stat programmed titration unit. For each trial, take 1 g of formulation into a thermostated response vessel and disperse in 18 ml of digestion media (50 mM Trizma maleate, 150 mM NaCl, 5 mM $CaCl_2 \cdot 2H_2O$, pH 7.5) having 5 mM NaTC (sodium taurocholate) and 1.25 mM PC (phosphatidyl choline). At that point, set the pH with 7.5 with 0.1 M NaOH. Begin digestion tests by the extension of 1 ml of pancreatin extract and maintain the mix at 37°C with continuous stirring. Utilize the pH-Stat programmed titration unit to keep up pH at 7.5±0.05 by titrating with 0.1 M NaOH. Record titrant volume at a predetermined time. The level of lipid digested is measured by calculating free unsaturated fats, which equivalents to the measure of consumed NaOH, which is given in **Equation 2**.

$$\text{Digestion percentage} = n_{FFA}(C_{NaOH} \times V_{NaOH}) \times M_{lipid} \times 100 \ldots.\text{Equation 2 } m_{lipid} \times 2 \qquad \textbf{(2)}$$

Where, n_{FFA} = numbers of free acids produced which are multiple of V_{NaOH} and C_{NaOH}, M_{lipid} = molecular weight of lipid, m_{lipid} = total mass of lipid, C_{NaOH} = concentration of NaOH consumed for titration, V_{NaOH} = volume of titrant NaOH used [35].

In Vitro Drug Release Assessment

This examination is performed to consider the drug discharge performance of preparation from the LCP around oil droplets utilizing a dialysis bag. Analysis of drug discharge is carried out through altered dispersion cells in 200 ml buffer media of pH 6.4. Take 1g of SMEDDS in a boiling tube. The two sides of this tube are open. Tie one part of the tube with a cellophane layer and plunge in a recepticle underneath. Bolster the upper side of the compartment, the stirrer is accustomed to mixing in estimating glass and draw test back after adequate time interims in a straight position and examine by the UV-spectrophotometer [36].

Thermodynamic Stability Study

This is done to assess the phase division and the impact of temperature deviation on SMEDDS formulation. Dilute SMEDDS with a liquid medium, centrifuge at 15,000 rpm for 15 min. and afterward watch outwardly for phase partition. Further formulation is kept to freeze-thaw cycles (-200°C for two days and +400°C for two days) and watched for phase separation [36, 37].

Permeability Study

For determination of improvement in bioavailability of preparation, one must need to carry out *in vitro* or *ex vivo* examination. For this, an isolated and perfused organ system needs to be utilized. Various methods are available for these.

The first one is, *In Situ* **Single-Pass Perfusion Technique** (SPIP), in which perfusion solution is passed *via* jejunum and these conditions gave *in vivo* environment. This strategy is helps to find out the exact retention mechanism that is active/passive/carrier-mediated retention.

Penetrability factor is dictated by computing the measure of drug which isn't assimilated in the intestine. The second method is **Everted sac** strategy in which a little piece of the intestine (2-4 cm) is knotted toward one side and everted utilizing a glass rod or thread. The method is utilized for determining dynamic parameters. For example, in the existence of sensitive recognition methods, radiolabelled drug transport over the intestine and *via* epithelial cells can be investigated. This strategy is appropriate for the determination of retention at diverse locations in small intestine and assessing the first-pass breakdown of xenobiotics in intestinal epithelial cells. The restriction of this procedure is that muscularis mucosa is available, which is normally not evacuated from everted sac formulations. Because of this reason, this strategy isn't favored for precise conclusions.

The third method is **Diffusion cell** strategy in which dispersion over a little piece of intestine or some other tissue (rectal, skin, buccal, lung, gastric) is examined utilizing the media with particular pH and temperature circumstances. On both sides of the diffusion membrane, the buffer solution is endlessly gassed with carbogen [38].

CONSENT FOR PUBLICATION

Not applicable.

CONFLICT OF INTEREST

The author declares no conflict of interest, financial or otherwise.

ACKNOWLEDGEMENTS

Declared none.

REFERENCES

[1]   Sachan R, Khatri K, Kasture SB. Self-emulsifying drug delivery system a novel approach for enhancement of Bioavailability. Int J Pharm Tech Res 2010; 2(3): 1738-45.

[2]   Yadav SK, Parvez N, Sharma PK. An insight to self-emulsifying drug delivery systems, their applications and importance in novel drug delivery. J Sci Invest Res 2014; 3(2): 273-81.

[3]   Gahlawat N, Verma R, Kaushik D. Recent developments in self-microemulsifying drug delivery system: An overview. Asian J Pharm 2019; 13(2): 59-72.

[4]   Jannin V, Musakhanian J, Marchaud D. Approaches for the development of solid and semi-solid lipid-based formulations. Adv Drug Deliv Rev 2008; 60(6): 734-46.
[http://dx.doi.org/10.1016/j.addr.2007.09.006] [PMID: 18045728]

[5]   Patel ND, Patel KV, Panchal LA, Shukla AK, Shelat PK. An emerging technique for poorly soluble drugs: Self-emulsifying drug delivery system. Int J Pharm Biol Arch 2011; 2(2): 621-9.

[6]   Verma R, Mittal V, Kaushik D. Self-microemulsifying drug delivery system: A vital approach for bioavailability enhancement. Int J Chemtech Res 2017; 10(7): 515-28.

[7]   Shukla JB, Koli AR, Ranch KM, Parikh RK. Self-micro emulsifying drug delivery system. Int J Pharm Pharm Sci 2010; 1(2): 13-33.

[8]   Pujara ND. Self-emulsifying drug delivery system: A novel approach. Int J Curr Pharm Res 2012; 4(2): 18-23.

[9]   Shaji J, Jadhav D. Newer approaches to self-emulsifying drug delivery system. Int J Pharm Pharm Sci 2010; 2(1): 37-42.

[10]   Sebastain G, Rajasree PH, George J, Gowda DV. Self-microemulsifying drug delivery systems (SMEEDS) as a potential drug delivery system-novel applications and future perspectives: A review. Int J Pharm 2016; 6: 105-10.

[11]   Wadhwa J, Nair A, Kumria R. Self-emulsifying therapeutic system: a potential approach for delivery of lipophilic drugs. Braz J Pharm Sci 2011; 47(3): 447-65.
[http://dx.doi.org/10.1590/S1984-82502011000300003]

[12]   Sarpal K, Pawar YB, Bansal AK. Self-emulsifying drug delivery systems: A strategy to improve oral bioavailability. Int J Curr Pharm Res 2010; 11(3): 42-55.

[13]   Verma R, Kaushik D. *In vitro* lipolysis as a tool for establishment of *IVIVC* for lipid based drug delivery systems. Curr Drug Deliv 2019; 16(8): 688-97.
[http://dx.doi.org/10.2174/1567201816666190620115716] [PMID: 31250755]

[14]   Sanghi DK, Tiwle R. A review on (SMEDDS) self micro-emulsifying drug delivery system. Int J Pharma Dev Tech 2015; 5(1): 20-6.

[15]   Kalamkar P, Pawar K, Baddi H, Thawkar B, Yevale R, Kale M. A Review on Self Micro Emulsifying Drug Delivery System (SMEDDS). Int J Pharma Pharm Res 2016; 6(3): 361-73.

[16]   Lalwani JT, Thakkar VT, Patel HV. Enhancement of solubility and oral bioavailability of ezetimibe by a novel solid self nano-emulsifying drug delivery system (SNEDDS). Int J Pharm Pharm Sci 2013; 5(3): 513-22.

[17]   Wagh MP, Singh PK, Chaudhari CS, Khairnar DA. Solid self-emulsifying drug delivery system: Preparation techniques and dosage forms. Int J Biopharm 2014; 5(2): 101-8.

[18]   Talele SG, Gudsoorkar VR. Novel approaches for solidification of SMEDDS. Int J Pharma Bio Sci 2016; 15: 90-101.

[19]   Mahapatra AK, Murthy PN, Swadeep B, Swain RP. Self-emulsifying drug delivery systems (SEDDS): An update from formulation development to therapeutic strategies. Int J Pharm Tech Res 2014; 6(2): 546-68.

[20]   Padia N, Shukla A, Shelat P. Development and characterization of fenofibrate self-microemulsifying drug delivery system (SMEDDS) for bioavailability enhancement. Bull Pharm Res 2015; 5(2): 59-69.

[21]   Gupta S, Kesarla R, Omri A. Formulation strategies to improve the bioavailability of poorly absorbed drugs with special emphasis on self-emulsifying systems 2013.
[http://dx.doi.org/10.1155/2013/848043]

[22] Verma R, Kaushik D. Design and optimization of candesartan loaded self-nanoemulsifying drug delivery system for improving its dissolution rate and pharmacodynamic potential 2020.
[http://dx.doi.org/10.1080/10717544.2020.1760961]

[23] Date AA, Nagarsenker MS. Design and evaluation of self-nanoemulsifying drug delivery systems (SNEDDS) for cefpodoxime proxetil. Int J Pharm 2007; 329(1-2): 166-72.
[http://dx.doi.org/10.1016/j.ijpharm.2006.08.038] [PMID: 17010543]

[24] Agrawal S, Giri TK, Tripathi DK, Alexander A. A review on novel therapeutic strategies for the enhancement of solubility for hydrophobic drugs through lipid and surfactant based self micro emulsifying drug delivery system: a novel approach. Am J Drug Disc Dev 2012; 2(4): 143-83.
[http://dx.doi.org/10.3923/ajdd.2012.143.183]

[25] Gershanik T, Benita S. Self-dispersing lipid formulations for improving oral absorption of lipophilic drugs. Eur J Pharm Biopharm 2000; 50(1): 179-88.
[http://dx.doi.org/10.1016/S0939-6411(00)00089-8] [PMID: 10840200]

[26] Sapra K, Sapra A, Singh SK, Kakkar S. Self-emulsifying drug delivery system: A tool in solubility enhancement of poorly soluble drugs. Indo Global J Pharm Sci 2012; 2(3): 313-32.

[27] Pouton CW. Self-emulsifying drug delivery systems: assessment of the efficiency of emulsification. Int J Pharm 1985; 27(2-3): 335-48.
[http://dx.doi.org/10.1016/0378-5173(85)90081-X]

[28] Kim JY, Ku YS. Enhanced absorption of indomethacin after oral or rectal administration of a self-emulsifying system containing indomethacin to rats. Int J Pharm 2000; 194(1): 81-9.
[http://dx.doi.org/10.1016/S0378-5173(99)00367-1] [PMID: 10601687]

[29] Parmar B, Patel U, Bhimani B, Sanghavi K, Patel G, Daslaniya D. SMEDDS: A dominant dosage form which improve bioavailability. Am J PharmTech Res 2012; 2(4): 54-72.

[30] Verma R, Mittal V, Kaushik D. Quality based design approach for improving oral bioavailability of valsartan loaded SMEDDS and study impact of lipolysis on the drug diffusion. Drug Deliv Lett 2018; 8(2): 130-9.
[http://dx.doi.org/10.2174/2210303108666180313141956]

[31] Agarwal V, Alayoubi A, Siddiqui A, Nazzal S. Powdered self-emulsified lipid formulations of meloxicam as solid dosage forms for oral administration. Drug Dev Ind Pharm 2012; 3(4): 1-9.
[PMID: 23072611]

[32] Patel PA, Chaulang GM, Akolkotkar A, Mutha SS, Hardikar SR, Bhosale AV. Self-emulsifying drug delivery system: A review. Res J Pharm and Technol 2008; 1(4): 313-23.

[33] Pattewar SKS, Pandey V, Sharma S. Self microemulsifying drug delivery system: A lipid-based drug delivery system. Int J Pharm Sci Res 2016; 7(2): 443-52.

[34] Janković J, Djekic L, Dobričić V, Primorac M. Evaluation of critical formulation parameters in design and differentiation of self-microemulsifying drug delivery systems (SMEDDSs) for oral delivery of aciclovir. Int J Pharm 2016; 497(1-2): 301-11.
[http://dx.doi.org/10.1016/j.ijpharm.2015.11.011] [PMID: 26611669]

[35] Khamkar GS. Self micro-emulsifying drug delivery system (SMEDDS) o/w microemulsion for BCS Class II drugs: An approach to enhance an oral bioavailability. Int J Pharm Pharm Sci 2011; 3(3): 1-3.

[36] Ghosh PK, Majithiya RJ, Umrethia ML, Murthy RS. Design and development of microemulsion drug delivery system of acyclovir for improvement of oral bioavailability. AAPS PharmSciTech 2006; 7(3): 77.
[http://dx.doi.org/10.1208/pt070377] [PMID: 17025257]

[37] Khedekar K, Mittal S. Self-emulsifying drug delivery system: A review. Int J Pharm Sci Res 2013; 4(12): 4494-506.

[38] Li Y, Zhang B, Liu M, *et al.* Further study of influence of *Panax notoginseng* on intestinal absorption

characteristics of triptolide and tripterine in Rats with *Tripterygium wilfordii*. Pharmacogn Mag 2018; 14(53): 95-102.
[http://dx.doi.org/10.4103/pm.pm_67_17] [PMID: 29576708]

CHAPTER 7

Solid-SMEDDS: Techniques of Solidification and Recent Advancements

Ravinder Verma[1], Deepak Kaushik[1], Parijat Pandey[2,*] and Pawan Jalwal[2]

[1] *Department of Pharmaceutical Sciences, Maharshi Dayanand University, Rohtak (Haryana), 124001, India*

[2] *Shri Baba Mastnath Institute of Pharmaceutical Sciences and Research, Baba Mastnath University, Rohtak (Haryana), 124001, India*

Abstract: From the point of view of dosage forms, S-SEDDS represents the solid dose formulation with self-emulsification features. The S-SEDDS becomes the focal point when adding liquid or semisolid SE components into powders or nanoparticles through various solidification strategies, such as adsorption to solid carriers, spray drying, spray cooling, supercritical liquid-based technique, melt extrusion, nanoparticle technology, *etc.* S-SMEDDS offers various benefits, such as diminishing the threat of interaction of the SMEDDS ingredients with the shell of the capsule. Immediate or controlled-release formulations can be formulated, relying upon the decision of the powder ingredient to be incorporated in the formulation; SE granules or pellets diminish the rate of the gastric emptying time and smooth entry in the gut, which generally leads to less threat of dosage fluctuations. Various types of S-SMEDDS include SE solid dispersions, SE tablets, SE enteric-coated dry emulsion, SE beads, SE sustained-release microspheres, SE nanoparticles, SE mouth dissolving film, SE floating dosage form, positively charged SMEDDS, self-double-emulsifying drug delivery system, supersaturatable SMEDDS, and so on. While lecithin-linker SEFs, sponges carrying SMEDDS, herbal SMEDDS and SE phospholipid suspension are novel S-SMEDDS. Different issues are related to the solidification strategies, such as the quantity of solidifying ingredients, the release rate of the drug, degradation of drug amid solidifying procedure, difficulty in content uniformity, decrease in drug loading limit and the probability of remaining solvents amid granulation and so on. In this chapter, an attempt has been made to highlight the various methods for solidifying SMEDDS, their issues and types of Solid-SMEDDS.

Keywords: Nanoparticles, Self-double-emulsifying drug delivery system techniques, SE pellets, SE mouth dissolving films, SE phospholipid suspension, Solid self-microemulsifying drug delivery system.

----
* **Corresponding author Parijat Pandey:** Shri Baba Mastnath Institute of Pharmaceutical Sciences and Research, Baba Mastnath University, Rohtak (Haryana), 124001, India; Tel: +91-9996233398; E-mail: parijatpandey98@gmail.com

SOLID SELF-EMULSIFYING DRUG DELIVERY SYSTEM

SEDDS can occur in solid or liquid dosage forms. These are generally limited to liquid forms as their numerous ingredients do not remain solids at ambient temperature. Known benefits of the solid dosage formulation have been widely studied, as they have evolved as more powerful options to liquid SEDDS with the time. The solid dosage forms of SEDDS represent solid dose formulations which have features of self-emulsification. Their focal point is the addition of liquid/semisolid SE components into powders/nanoparticles by various solidification strategies. There are various approaches for the solidification of SMEDDS which are shown in Fig. (**1**). Such as nanoparticle/powder, which alludes to self-emulsifying solid dispersions/dry emulsions/nanoparticles, and are converted into other solid dosage formulation or filled into capsules which are known as SE capsules. These are generally incorporated/filled into capsules without any solidifying ingredient. S-SEDDS are a blend of solid dosage formulation and SEDDS. Several features of S-SEDDS (*e.g.* ingredients determination, specificity and evaluation) are the relating features of both SEDDS and solid dosage formulation.

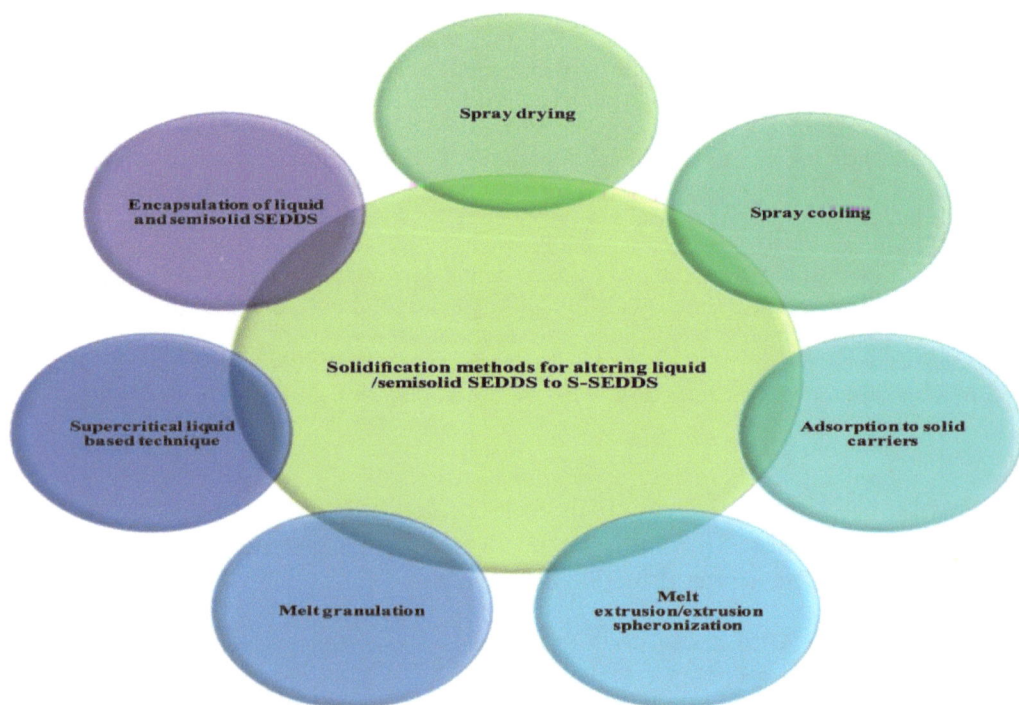

Fig. (1). Various approaches for solidification of SMEDDS.

The evaluations of SE pellets include self-emulsification time, as well as friability, surface texture, *etc*. In 1990s, these were generally in the shape of SE capsule, SE solid dispersion and dry emulsion. However, other solid SE dosage formulation has been developed such as SE pellets/tablets, SE microspheres/nanoparticles and SE suppositories/ implants [1 - 3].

Various benefits of oral solid dosage formulations are [4, 5]:

(a) Less manufacturing charges.

(b) Ease to process variables.

(c) Elevated stability and reproducibility.

(d) Improved patient compliance.

Solidification Methods for Altering Semisolid/Liquid Self-emulsifying Drug Delivery System to S-SEDDS

Filling of the capsule with semisolid/liquid SEFs

Capsule filling is the least difficult and the most widely recognized innovation for encapsulating the semisolid/liquid SEFs for oral administration. A four steps method is used for semisolid preparations [6]:

(i) Warming the semisolid ingredients to not less than 20°C, over the melting temperature

(ii) Joining of the dynamic substances (along with mixing)

(iii) Filling the container with liquid blend and

(iv) Cooling at ambient temperature.

For liquid preparations, it includes a two-stage method: filling of semisolid formulation into the capsules by settling the crown and body of the capsule using micro-spray. The advancement in Capsule Innovation Continuing, and liquid OROS (Alza Corporation) has been proposed for controlled delivery of insoluble drug compounds or peptides. The system relies upon osmotic pressure is liquid SEFs. It involves an osmotic layer, which stretches out to avoid contact with the aqueous phase and pumps the drug formulation through a hole/orifice in the hard or flexible container. An essential consideration that should be kept in mind during capsule filling is to identify that how compatible the ingredients and the container shell are. The compatibility of semisolid/liquid hydrophobic ingredients with hard capsules was recorded by Cole *et al*. The benefits of container filling are straightforwardness in collecting; propriety for low-estimations, exceptionally potent drugs and high drug loading potential [7].

Spray Drying

Generally, this strategy includes the development of preparation by amalgamation of surfactants, lipids, solid carriers, drug and solubilize the amalgamate before spray drying. Atomization of solubilized liquid preparation into a spray of globules is carried out. The globules are brought into a drying chamber, in which the volatile phase evaporates, dry particles are prepared under controlled air flow and temperature conditions. Particles like these can also be organized into capsules or tablets. The temperature, the atomizer, the drying chamber pattern and the most appropriate air flow are picked up by the drying attributes of the item and the desired specifications of the powder [8].

Čerpnjak *et al.,* 2015 developed naproxen loaded tablets and minitablets employing this technique. They found a low dissolution profile of naproxen from tablets and minitablets compared to the liquid and solid SMEDDS [9].

Bhandari *et al.* designed artemether-lumefantrine-loaded S-SMEDDS employing this technique with Neusilin US2. A high-dose combination of solid SMEDDS was capable of maintaining plasma concentration of lumefantrine above the minimum effective concentration for ≈4 days. Solid SMEDDS containing low-, medium- and high-dose combinations of artemether and lumefantrine are more effective than marketed tablets [10].

Kim *et al.* 2015 developed dutasteride-loaded solid supersaturatable SMEDDS using this technique with Aerosil 200 colloidal silica. They found that solid SMEDDS/aerosil 200/Soluplus microparticles had greater bioavailability (6.8 and 5.0-times) higher C_{max} and AUC values, respectively than that of the equivalent physical mixture [11].

Spray Cooling

Spray cooling is also known as spray congealing. It is a procedure whereby the molten formulation is showered into a cooling chamber. The liquid droplet solidifies and recrystallizes into round solid particles when molten formulation came in contact with the cool air. Solidified particles fall over the base of the heap and are likewise assembled like a fine powder. Then, the fine powder might be utilized for designing solid dosage formulations like tablets or powder. Various kinds of apparatus are handy to atomize the mixture of liquid and to create beads. Some of these include rotary pressure, two-fluid or ultrasonic atomizers [12].

Adsorption to Solid Carriers

The liquid SEDDS can be easily adsorbed onto free streaming powders that have tremendous surface area, suitable for adsorbing huge amounts of lipidic components. This is feasible either by mixing liquid SEDDS and adsorbent in a blender or by simple physical mixing. The consequent powders can be either filled into capsules or can be converted into tablets after the addition of suitable ingredients. These carriers may be micro-porous inorganic compounds, high surface range colloidal inorganic compounds or cross-linked polymers. Classes of solid adsorbents used are silicates, talc, crospovidone, cross-linked polymethyl methacrylate and so on. Cross-linked polymers make an ideal situation to maintain drug dissolution and help with backing off drug precipitation. Oral solid SMEDDS of heparin and gentamicin were got ready using three types of adsorbents: microporous calcium silicate, magnesium aluminometa silicate and silicon dioxide [13].

Bhagwat *et al.,* 2012 developed solid SMEDDS with this technique using acrysol EL 135, polysorbate 80, PEG 400 and aerosil 200. They concluded that S-SMEDDS resulted in significantly higher dissolution rate as compared to the pure drug. *Ex vivo* intestinal permeability investigation demonstrated that diffusion of drug was considerably higher from S-SMEDDS than that of suspension [14].

Tamboli *et al.* designed diacerein loaded solid SMEDDS with this technique using oleic acid, tween 80, polyethylene glycol 200 and neusilin US2. Reconstitution properties of formulation demonstrated spontaneous microemulsification with globule size 0.271 μm and −16.18 mV zeta potential. From the results of *in vitro* dissolution testing, it was found that the release of diacerein was significantly increased as compared with pure drug [15].

Melt Granulation

This is a method in which powder agglomeration is obtained by the consolidation of a cover that melts or mollifies at moderately low temperatures. As a 'one-step' operation, melt granulation proposes benefits from traditional wet granulation because of the fluid extension and drying stage are avoided. The essential factors that control the granulation methodology are impeller speed, time of mixing, molecule size of drug and the carrier thickness. A broad assortment of solid and semisolid lipids can be used as a meltable carrier. Gelucire, a mixture of concentrations got from the mixes of mono-/di-/tri-glycerides and PEG esters of unsaturated fats can also extend the rate of disintegration differentiated and PEG for improving its SE property. Other LBFs investigations for melt granulation to make solid SES contain lecithin, glycerides or polysorbates. This process is normally used for adsorbing SEFs onto basically silica and magnesium aluminometa silicate [13].

Kishore *et al.,* 2015 developed Atorvastatin loaded S-SMEDDS using this technique with coconut oil and IPM as oily phase; Tween 80 as a surfactant; PEG 400 and glycerin. They found that SMEDDS (1:3) with solid carrier demonstrated more drug release due to their less particle size. The solid SMEDDS showed improved dissolution profiles. Transformation of the solid-state of the drug in formulation resulting in improved solubility [16].

Vadlamudi *et al.,* 2017 designed bosentan loaded solid SMEDDS and found that solid SMEDDS had high-dissolution profiles than pure bosentan due to modification in the crystalline structure of the drug upon microemulsification [17].

Melt Extrusion/Extrusion Spheronization

This is a soluble free technique that grants high drug loading (60%) and good content consistency. Extrusion is a strategy of transforming a crude compound with plastic features into a thing of uniform shape and thickness by obliging it through a pass under thermo-controlled conditions, product flow rate and pressure conditions. The approximate size of the resulting spheroids will be chosen by the type of extruder opening. This process is ordinarily utilized in the pharmaceutical industry to formulate consistently assessed spheroids (pellets).

The extrusion–spheronization method involves these means dry mixing of excipients and API to achieve a homogeneous powder, wet massing with the binder, extrusion into a spaghetti-like extrudate, spheronization from the extrudate to spheroids of uniform size; drying; separating to attain the pined for measure dispersion and then covering (non-compulsory). The relative quantity of SEFs and water had a sufficient impact on the expulsion force, globule size, time of disintegration and the surface texture of pellets. Various investigations recommended that most of these SEFs can be solidified by expulsion spheronization which contains 42% of the dry pellet weight. In general, the higher the water level, the more drawn out the breaking downtime. It has been confirmed that SEFs holding wet mass with an extensive variety of rheological features can be handled, yet a solitary rheological factor can't be utilized to give an entire assessment of how well it may be set up by extrusion–spheronization. By using this technique, diazepam and progesterone loaded SE pellets and bi-layered SE pellets have been formulated [8].

Silva *et al.,* 2018 developed carvedilol loaded solid SMEDDS by blending lipidic mixture and HPMCAS with a twin-screw hot melt extruder. They found that extrudates developed with the lowest drug concentration, highest temperature and recirculation time resulted in a complete and quick drug discharge in pH 6.8 giving rise to small and uniform microemulsion globules [18].

Supercritical Liquid-based Technique

Lipids might be utilized as a part of this strategy either to coat the drug molecules or creating solid dispersion. For natural reasons, the ideal supercritical liquid of decision is supercritical CO_2. The illustration incorporates controlled discharge applications employing glyceryl trimyristate and stearoylpolyoxylglycerides [19]. All the more particularly, they offer the accompanying points of interest:

1. They diminish the threat of incompatibility of the ingredients with the capsule shell, along these lines offering stability enhancement because of the lessened danger of chemical degradation and microbial growth, suggesting an expanded period of usability.

2. They can be formulated as immediate or controlled release preparations relying upon the decision of the powder ingredient with which the SMEDDS is formulated

3. They avoid severe meting out necessities because these are solid dosage forms.

4. They offer accuracy in dose uniformity.

5. They are effortlessly transferred and stored.

6. Manufacturing cost is impressively low compared with liquid container filling.

7. SE coarse powders, granules and pellets have excellent flowability, permitting quick and reproducible capsule or die-filling, empowering high production rates.

8. SE granules or pellets, specifically, being various unit dose forms offer therapeutic preferences that are feature for these dosage forms. They advance diminishment of the variety of the gastric emptying time, the smooth entry in the gut and generally less threat of dosage fluctuations.

9. More significantly, investigations have demonstrated that the release of progesterone in dogs from SE pellets was proportionate to intake of liquid microemulsion [20 - 22].

Issues Related to the Solidification Strategies

There are various issues related to solidification strategies. These issues take account for the following:

1. Quantity of solidifying ingredients may control the release rate of the drug

2. Degradation of drug amid solidifying procedure

3. Difficulty in guaranteeing content uniformity

4. Blockage of spray nozzles because of oil content in spray drying strategy

5. Nature of the ingredients used may affect the drug retention

6. Lessening in drug loading limit

7. Possibility of irreversible phase partition on reconstitution

8. Possibility of remaining solvents which is utilized amid granulation [23].

Ways to Deal with the Problems of Solidification Strategies

With a specific end goal to lessen the quantity of solidifying ingredients required for conversion of SMEDDS into solid dosage formulation, a gelled SMEDDS is produced. For this, LBFs colloidal silicon dioxide (Aerosil 200) was chosen as a gelling agent, which performed the dual function of diminishing the quantity of essential solidifying ingredients and helping in slowing down the drug discharge profile. After oral intake of capsules containing ordinary liquid SE formulations, it converts into emulsion droplets and in this way, it disperses in the GIT to achieve retention at the target site. Be that as it may, if irreversible phase separation of the emulsion occurs, an alteration of drug retention can't be normal.

(a) For avoiding this risk, sodium dodecyl sulfate is incorporated into the SE formulation.

(b) With comparable reason, the supersaturatable SMEDDS was outlined, using a minute quantity of HPMC (or different polymers) in the formulation to prevent precipitation of the drug by creating and achieving a supersaturation condition of *in vivo*. These systems had a lessened quantity of surfactant that results in the lessening of GI side effects [24].

Various Advancements of S-SMEDDS

Traditional liquid SMEDDS has various limitations in the manufacturing process such as high manufacturing costs, difficulty in usage, physical incompatibility issues with shells of soft gelatin and storage issues. Physical incompatibility of liquid SMEDDS can be prevented by filling S-SMEDDS in the capsules. In the case of semisolid excipients, after melting and cooling, it is filled into capsules; its contents solidify at the normal temperature [25]. Various advancements of S-

SMEDDS are shown in Fig. (**2**) and discussed below:

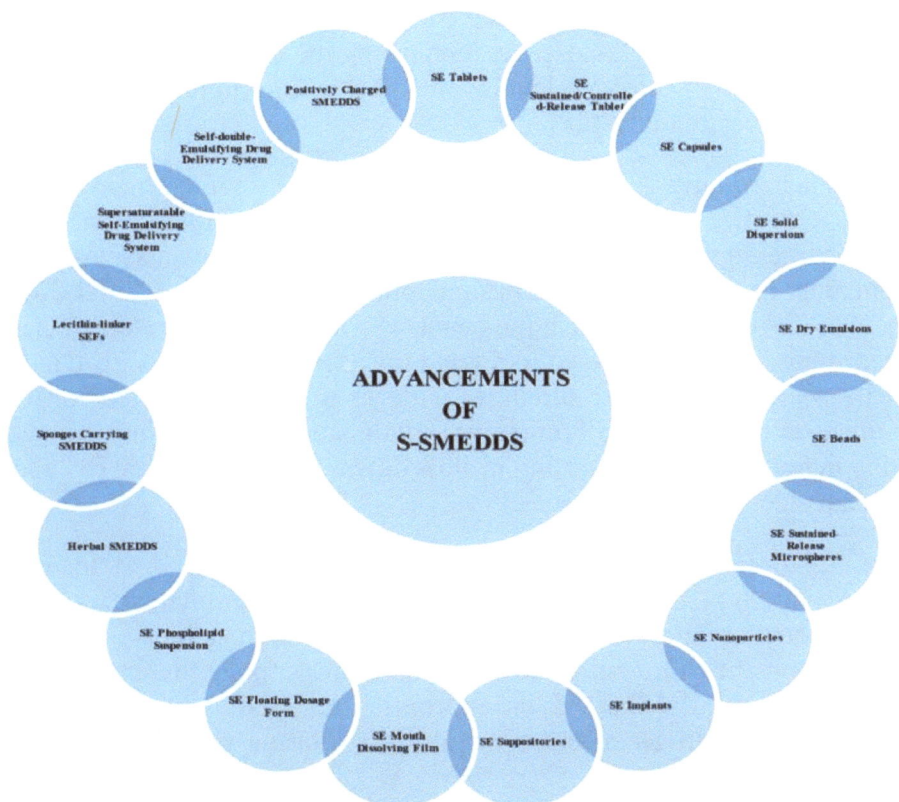

Fig. (2). Various advancements of S-SMEDDS.

SE Tablets

Tablets are solid dosage forms that generally consist of drugs and ingredients in powder, crystalline or granular form with or without diluents, formulated either by molding or compression process. Their ease of convenience and various types results in achieving their widespread usage [26].

Eutectic based self-emulsifying tablets were formulated by Nazzal *et al.* which inhibit irreversible precipitation of the drug within the formulation. A combination of drug and appropriate semisolid oil was used in the preparation. The melting point depression method was employed in which the oil phase contained drug and formulation melts at body temperature producing nano globules of emulsion. During the formulation of these tablets maltodextrin, modified povidone and MCC were employed as carriers [27].

SE Sustained/Controlled-Release Tablets

Controlled-release (CR) formulations have been introduced into drug therapy for reducing the number of single-dose/day, enhancing the compliance of patient and decline fluctuations of plasma levels, thus achieving improved therapeutic efficiency and lower toxicity [28].

Nazzal and Khan have investigated the impact of various manufacturing parameters (Quantity of colloidal silicates-X_1, mixing timing of magnesium stearate-X_2 and compression force-X_3) on hardness and rate of dissolution from the formulation. Face-centered cubic design optimized conditions (X_1 = 1.06%, X_2 = 2 min, X = 1670 kgf) to diminish the quantity of solidifying ingredients needed for transforming of SEDDS into solid dosage forms. Patil *et al.,* designed a gelled SEDDS by selecting colloidal silicon dioxide as a gelling agent for oil-based formulations, that fulfills dual functions, diminishing the measure of needed solidifying ingredients and supporting in slow down of drug discharge (by altering the molecular size of MCC) [27].

Nazzal *et al.,* designed ubiquinone loaded self-nanoemulsified tablet dosage formulation. Firstly, self-nanoemulsion system was formulated which was absorbed on granular ingredients and then compressed to the tablets dosage form. For the development of a controlled-discharge matrix, polyethylene oxide was used which successfully showed its appropriateness. SE tablets consistently maintained a greater drug concentration in blood plasma when compared with simple tablets [29].

Various potent drugs have less oral bioavailability because of their very less aqueous solubility or pre-systemic metabolism. Carvedilol drug belongs to the BCS IV class which has pre-systemic metabolism. SE tablets are of extraordinary usefulness in avoiding adverse effects, as revealed by Schwarz in the patent. The novel self-emulsifying osmotic pump tablet (SEOPT) loaded with carvedilol has numerous focal points such as steady plasma concentrations, controllable drug discharge rate and bioavailability of 156.78% when compared with the marketed tablet. The inclusion of hydrophobic NSAIDS into SE tablets may boost their penetration potential through GI mucosa, potentially diminishing the bleeding in GI. In these investigations, the SE system contained glycerol monolaurate and tyloxapol TM [30, 31].

SE Capsules

Capsules are solid dosage forms that enclose one or more drugs within a special small shell or container generally formulated from appropriate gelatin. Depending upon the type of preparation, the capsule shell may be hard or soft.

Oral administration of SE capsules enhances patient compliance when compared with the parental route. For example, low molecular weight heparin (LMWH) utilized for curing venous thrombo-embolism is clinically used only *via* parental route. Ito *et al.*, developed its oral therapy. LMWH dispersed in SMEDDS and afterward, mixture solidified to powders by utilizing adsorbents such as FloriteTM RE, NeusilinTM US2 and SylysiaTM 320. Eventually, hard capsules were filled with these solids. In another study, SE tablets of gentamicin are in medical utilization, while it was restricted to administer as injectable or topical dosage forms earlier [32].

S-SMEDDS are filled into capsule shells that are prepared by various techniques. Capsule filling is the least difficult and the most well-known innovation for the encapsulation of liquid, semisolid or solid SE preparations. The benefits of capsule filling are ease of development, suitability for very potent low-dose drugs and high drug loading potential. It involves a two-step procedure for liquid preparations which includes: filling preparation into the capsules [23].

SE Solid Dispersions

An amorphous solid dispersion (ASD) results from a formulation technique in which the drug is molecularly dispersed in a polymer [33].

Gelucire 44/14 and Gelucire 50/02 are employed for this purpose because these are semisolid excipients and can be directly filled into capsules in a molten state. Processing and stability issues associated with solid dispersions were reduced due to the availability of self-dispersing waxy semisolid ingredients. These ingredients can probably expand the digestion of inadequately water-soluble drugs to early utilized PEG solid dispersions and may likewise be filled specifically into hard gelatin capsules in the liquid state, in this manner obviating the former requirement for milling and blending before filling. SE ingredients like Gelucire 44/14, Gelucire 150/02, labrasol, transcutol and TPGS have been generally employed in this area. Assimilation of the drugs is enhanced when Gelucire is employed as a carrier because Gelucire has high surface activity [34].

SE Dry Emulsions

These are powdered solid dosage formulations which instantly emulsify by incorporation of water in the formulation. They can be obtained by emulsifiable glass systems, freeze-drying and spray drying. A newly designed enteric-coated dry emulsion formulation is the most exciting discovery in this field. This formulation consists of amlodipine with dextrin as a carrier for oral deliverance of peptide and protein drugs by Toorisaka *et al.* [35].

Cui *et al.,* spread liquid o/w emulsion on flat glass, afterward dried and triturated to powders for developing dry emulsions. Freeze drying of o/w emulsion with amorphous cryoprotectants was explained by Bamba *et al.* [36].

Vyas *et al.,* prepared dry emulsion of griseofulvin utilizing mannitol as cryoprotectant. Corveleyn *et al.,* investigated the parameter that incorporation of amorphous cryoprotectants influences the cooling rate. Both of these have the best stabilizing impacts, while heat treatment prior to thawing diminishes the stabilizing impacts on the preparation of lyophilized dry emulsion tablets [37].

Myers and Shively developed solid-state glass emulsions. In this method, the drug dissolved in vegetable oil was mixed with an aqueous solution of sucrose. Such emulsifiable glasses have the benefit that they exclude surfactant in the formulation and the surfactant is no more required. The dry foam was produced by rotator evaporation of mixture under vacuum. The emulsion was produced by the addition of these to this dry foam. Cyclosporin A was tried to deliver *via* this method. The technique of spray drying is more frequently employed in the formulation of dry emulsions. The o/w emulsion was prepared and then spray dried to eliminate the aqueous phase [38].

SE Beads

Porous polystyrene beads for delivering SEFs were used by Patil. The formulation is poured into microchannels of the bead through capillary action. Copolymerization of styrene and divinylbenzene is done to prepare the beads [39].

Self-emulsifying Pellets (SE pellets)

Oral pellets are also recognized to conquer poor and uneven GIT assimilation of drugs and have demonstrated the potential to decrease or remove food-effect. Thus, it seems highly appealing to merge the benefits of pellets with those of SETs by formulating this formulation.

Franceschinis *et al.* designed a new technique for the formulation of SE pellets by wet granulation using oil as a binder (mono and diglycerides), tween 80 and nimesulide. Binder solution contained a blend of oil and surfactant with water. The prepared binder solutions were sprayed onto the granules (prepared from MCC and lactose) to give pellets. *In vivo* investigations demonstrated considerable greater bioavailability with the pellets in contrast to the emulsions [40].

Wang *et al.* demonstrated large scale manufacturing of nitrendipine employing extrusion/ spheronization method for production of SE pellets from the liquid SEF to enhance oral assimilation. The liquid SEFs were solidified with adsorbents (porous silicon dioxide), MCC and lactose to create fine flowable powder [41].

SE Sustained-release Microspheres

Microspheres are spherical microparticles that can be used as drug carriers. The size of microspheres is in the micron range. Microspheres are mostly formed of biodegradable polymers. Their major benefit is their provision of stability for labile drugs that are easily degraded in the intestinal epithelium.

Quasi-emulsion-solvent-diffusion method was used to prepare sustained-release microspheres of zedoary turmeric oil using HPMC acetate succinate and aerosil 200 [42].

SE Nanoparticles

Solvent injection technique, sonication emulsion-diffusion-evaporation can be used for the development of SNEFs. Drug and excipients are melted together and injected into a non-solvent solution. Nanoparticles can be separated by centrifugation and lyophilization. Goat fat and tween 65 were used for the development of SNEFs. Glyceryl monooleate (GMO), having self-emulsifying feature was used for the preparation of paclitaxel nanoparticles with chitosan. Chitosan acts as bio-adhesive for nanoparticles, while 100% drug incorporation was attained due to the SE feature of GMO [12, 30].

SE Implants

Self-emulsified carmustine was added into PLGA water and utilized as an implant. SEDDS preparation decreased exposure of carmustine from aqueous media, its stability and shelf-life increased. This preparation contained tributyrin, cremophor RH 40, labrafil MC 1944 and carmustine [12].

SE Suppositories

Suppositories are dosage forms that are used to insert the drugs into cavities of the body. In the majority of cases, the rectum is used for the deliverance of drugs to blood circulation or local tissues [43].

C_6-C_{18} FA glycerol ester and C_6-C_8 FA macrogol esters were employed in the development of glycyrrhizin self-emulsifying suppositories. This Formulation reported good drug assimilation which is demonstrated by high plasma drug levels when delivered through the rectal/vaginal route [44].

SE Mouth Dissolving Film (SMMDF)

Mouth dissolving films (MDF) offers a well-situated way of dosing drugs to special population groups with swallowing problems such as pediatric, geriatric patients and the general population. These are the novel dosage forms that disintegrate and dissolve within the oral cavity. Intra-oral assimilation permits rapid onset of action and helps to avoid first-pass metabolism, thereby dropping the unit dose essential to produce desired therapeutic effect [45].

Xiao *et al.* developed SMMDF for indomethacin by fusing self-microemulsifying systems with solid carriers (MCC, low-substituted HPMC and hypromellose). They concluded that SMMDF is another promising dosage form, exhibiting remarkable attributes of accommodation, fast response and increment in oral bioavailability of PWS drugs [46].

SE Floating Dosage Form

The main issues regarding the low bioavailability are low solubility, pre-systemic metabolism and eradicate absorption of drugs throughout the GIT. The floating system increases the residence time of the drug in the stomach and develops prolonged-release forms. Furosemide drug is used for the development of the novel floating dosage formulation to improve its solubility by preparing SMEDDS, trailed by its adsorption onto a blend of high functionality ingredient, matrix-forming polymers (HPMC K4M and HPMC E50 LV) and an effervescent agent ($NaHCO_3$) to attain a buoyant matrix with a controlled discharge profile [42].

Positively Charged SMEDDS

A standout amongst the most common issues faced by the formulation researchers has been to discover strategies for enhancing the oral bioavailability of PWS drugs. This positively charged SEDDS is developed by using cationic lipids which increment in the bioavailability than those of the negatively charged. Example- Meloxicam positively charged SEDDS were formulated by utilizing (ethyl oleate, sunflower oil and arachis oil) as oil components, (oleylamine) as cationic lipid and (combination of tween 80 and span 80) as surfactants in the formulation [47].

Self-double-emulsifying Drug Delivery System (SDEDDS)

Double emulsions (water-in-oil-in-water) are produced instantly in SDEDDS which is mixed in the aqueous GI milieu. In SDEDDS, the drug is encapsulated in its internal phase. Pidotimod, a peptide-like drug of BCS IV class SDEDDS is formulated to enhance their oral assimilation [42].

Supersaturatable Self-emulsifying Drug Delivery System (S-SEDDS)

Supersaturation represents a potent technique for improving the assimilation by generating and maintaining a supersaturated condition in the intestine. These formulations have reduced the quantity of surfactant and polymeric precipitation inhibitor that helps in achieving a supersaturated state of the drug in the body. In comparison with SEDDS, S-SEDDS formulations can result in improved stability and low toxicity [48].

Higuchi *et al.,* proposed the potential of supersaturated drug formulations in the improvement of drug absorption. PVP and water-soluble cellulosic polymers such as HPMC, methylcellulose, hydroxyl propyl methylcellulose phthalate are helpful in creating a supersaturatable form with several PWS drugs. A high payload S-SEDDS was explored to enhance the oral bioavailability of silybin employing HPMC as a precipitation inhibitor [49].

Delivery of Nutraceuticals by Lecithin-linker SEFs

Lecithin-linker microemulsions are preparations that are formulated with soybean lecithin in combination with lipophilic (lipophilic linker) and hydrophilic (hydrophilic linkers) surfactant-like additives [50].

Chu *et al.,* evaluated the microemulsions formed by lecithin-linker. In their formulation, they blended soybean lecithin with a hydrophilic and lipophilic linker. Self-emulsification was created by lecithin-linker with b-sitosterol and β-carotene. In order to minimize or reduce the development of fluid precious stones, a grouping of the sorbitan monooleate and lipophilic linker was done by the inventors. Further, PEG-6-caprylic/capric glycerides, decaglyceryl caprylate/caprate and the hydrophilic linkers were grouped and expanded steadily until the formation of transparent microemulsions. The micro-emulsion so formed was clear, stable and single-phase, having a droplet size near 200 nm. Using pseudo-ternary stage charts to assess the procedure of dilution of microemulsion preconcentrates (the blends of oil, lecithin and linkers with practically no water) with FeSSIF (Fed-state simulated intestinal fluid), it was resolved that self-emulsification acquired when the early phases of the dilution produce single-phase microemulsions. The numerous stages are acquired to avoid those early stages; the emulsification produces unstable emulsions with substantial drop sizes. An *in vitro* permeability study was directed utilizing a Flow-Thru Dialyzer. Dialyzer chamber is used to isolate precarious emulsions [51].

Sponges Carrying SMEDDS

Nanosponge technology is a novel and rising technology which uses the targeted drug delivery system to discharge a drug in a controlled manner to the targeted site. Nanosponges are the type of encapsulating nanoparticles that encapsulate the drug molecule within the core by various techniques of association and they can be classified into encapsulating nanoparticles, complexing nanoparticles, conjugating nanoparticles. These are solid, insoluble in water and organic solvents. These can be fabricated as oral, parenteral, topical or inhalation dosage form [52].

Josef *et al.,* studied that SMEDDS make the solvency of lipophilic drugs, their fluid nature is one boundary to their wide application. Their addition in sponges made from a hydrophilic polymer is a new technique for the formulation of SMEDDS. The nanosponge structures concentrated on examining in electron microscopy and small-angle X-ray diffusing. The oil beads were dried and SMEDDS of 9 nm-sized objects in the dried sponges were found. The sponges were rehydrated in water and confirmation of the presence of SMEDDS in the rehydrated sponges was found. A model hydrophobicdrug, Nile red was used as a solvent in all dry and rehydrated sponges. SMEDDS containing Nile red discharged from the nanosponges at a rate that depends upon the drying technique. The water uptake of the nanosponges was found to be affected by the drying formulation. The blend of SMEDDS and sponges may be an approach to beat the drawbacks of every part independently, give a strong measurement structure for SMEDDS that can manage the arrival of drugs furthermore empower the usage of hydrophilic sponges for the conveyance of hydrophobic drug [53].

Herbal SMEDDS

SMEDDS gives the option of liquids filled a hard gelatin capsule for the herbal extract for developing stable and safe dosage forms. In various vehicles, solubility of the herbal extract was find out. For evaluation of the micro emulsification existence area pseudo ternary phase diagrams were drawn. The discharge rate of the herbal extract was studied using the dissolution method. Clarity, precipitation and particle size distribution parameters were assessed for characterization of the formulation. Based on results of solubility and phase diagram screening and formulation development were carried out. Warke *et al.,* used the optimized formulation contain 30% herbal extract, 40% cremophor RH 40 and 30% plurol oleique which give complete release in 10 min. by utilizing *in vitro* method of dissolution. SMEDDS successfully passed the stability study for 3 months under different conditions. SMEDDS seemed to be a fascinating way to deal with enhancement in solubility and ultimately bioavailability [54].

SE Phospholipid Suspension (SEPS)

SEPS has a large quantity of phospholipids that are capable to maintain the drug in solubilized form *in vivo* environment, which is necessary for bioavailability upgrading. Phospholipids are endogenous lipids that have sufficient *in vivo* emulsification potential. These need moderately less quantity of surfactant/co-surfactant due to which they are less toxic to health [23].

The most regular strategy of S-SMEDDS development is the spray drying strategy in which solid carriers are used such as dextran, gelatin, aerosol 200 and lactose. These are effectively utilized for the development of S-SMEDDS like telmisartan, simvastatin, dexibuprofen, docetaxel and so on with superior oral bioavailability. Agarwal *et al.,* developed SE powder of meloxicam by using simple trituration of liquid SMEDDS with a solid carrier in a ratio of 1:1 (mixture of silicon dioxide and magnesium aluminum silicate) in a mortar until a homogenous mixture was produced to prepare this. This S-SMEDDS formulation demonstrated superior bioavailability in beagle dogs when compared with marketed tablets dosage form. It is a cost-efficient method to formulate a variety of solid oral dosage forms of BCS II and IV class drugs defeating the drawbacks of the conventional liquid SMEDDS formulations. Be that as it may, certain features of S-SMEDDS such as oxidation of vegetable oils, physical aging concerned with glyceride and interaction of drug and ingredients must be well thought-out while formulating S-SMEDDS.

In an investigation, the drawbacks of S-SMEDDS were studies i-e: the strong adsorption and physical interaction of drug with the carriers which result in delay or partial discharge of the drug from the formulation. In the same investigation, IR SE tablets of ibuprofen were developed by using Fujicalin® (granulated dibasic calcium phosphate) which is an acid-soluble powdering carrier that facilitates the drug discharge process in the gastric, this suggested an advanced strategy to formulate IR S-SMEDDS [34].

CONSENT FOR PUBLICATION

Not applicable.

CONFLICT OF INTEREST

The author declares no conflict of interest, financial or otherwise.

ACKNOWLEDGEMENTS

Declared none.

REFERENCES

[1]   Attama AA, Nzekwe IT, Nnamani PO, Adikwu MU, Onugu CO. The use of solid self-emulsifying systems in the delivery of diclofenac. Int J Pharm 2003; 262(1-2): 23-8.
[http://dx.doi.org/10.1016/S0378-5173(03)00315-6] [PMID: 12927384]

[2]   Abdalla A, Mäder K. Preparation and characterization of a self-emulsifying pellet formulation. Eur J Pharm Biopharm 2007; 66(2): 220-6.
[http://dx.doi.org/10.1016/j.ejpb.2006.11.015] [PMID: 17196807]

[3]   Kreilgaard M. Influence of microemulsions on cutaneous drug delivery. Bulletin Technique Gattefosse. 2002: N (95); 79-100.
[http://dx.doi.org/10.1016/S0169-409X(02)00116-3]

[4]   Hoar TP, Shulman JH. University of Cambridge Nobel Laureates. England, UK 1943.

[5]   Yi T, Wan J, Xu H, Yang X. A new solid self-microemulsifying formulation prepared by spray-drying to improve the oral bioavailability of poorly water soluble drugs. Eur J Pharm Biopharm 2008; 70(2): 439-44.
[http://dx.doi.org/10.1016/j.ejpb.2008.05.001] [PMID: 18603415]

[6]   Beg S, Swain S, Singh HP, Patra ChN, Rao ME. Development, optimization, and characterization of solid self-nanoemulsifying drug delivery systems of valsartan using porous carriers. AAPS PharmSciTech 2012; 13(4): 1416-27.
[http://dx.doi.org/10.1208/s12249-012-9865-5] [PMID: 23070560]

[7]   Cole ET, Cadé D, Benameur H. Challenges and opportunities in the encapsulation of liquid and semi-solid formulations into capsules for oral administration. Adv Drug Deliv Rev 2008; 60(6): 747-56.
[http://dx.doi.org/10.1016/j.addr.2007.09.009] [PMID: 18096270]

[8]   Tang B, Cheng G, Gu JC, Xu CH. Development of solid self-emulsifying drug delivery systems: preparation techniques and dosage forms. Drug Discov Today 2008; 13(13-14): 606-12.
[http://dx.doi.org/10.1016/j.drudis.2008.04.006] [PMID: 18598917]

[9]   Čerpnjak K, Pobirk AZ, Vrečer F, Gašperlin M. Tablets and minitablets prepared from spray-dried SMEDDS containing naproxen. Int J Pharm 2015; 495(1): 336-46.
[http://dx.doi.org/10.1016/j.ijpharm.2015.08.099] [PMID: 26341323]

[10]   Bhandari S, Bhandari V, Sood J, *et al.* Improved pharmacokinetic and pharmacodynamic attributes of artemether-lumefantrine-loaded solid SMEDDS for oral administration. J Pharm Pharmacol 2017; 69(11): 1437-46.
[http://dx.doi.org/10.1111/jphp.12795] [PMID: 28809448]

[11]   Kim MS, Ha ES, Choo GH, Baek IH. Preparation and *in vivo* evaluation of a dutasteride-loaded solid-supersaturatable self-microemulsifying drug delivery system. Int J Mol Sci 2015; 16(5): 10821-33.
[http://dx.doi.org/10.3390/ijms160510821] [PMID: 25984604]

[12]   Mahapatra AK, Murthy PN, Swadeep B, Swain RP. Self-emulsifying drug delivery systems (SEDDS): An update from formulation development to therapeutic strategies. Int J Pharm Tech Res 2014; 6(2): 546-68.

[13]   Talele SG, Gudsoorkar VR. Novel approaches for solidification of SMEDDS. Int J Pharma Bio Sci 2016; 15: 90-101.

[14]   Bhagwat DA, D'Souza JI. Formulation and evaluation of solid self micro emulsifying drug delivery system using aerosil 200 as solid carrier. Int Curr Pharm J 2012; 1(12): 414-9.http://www.icpjonline.com/documents/Vol1Issue12/04.pdf
[http://dx.doi.org/10.3329/icpj.v1i12.12451]

[15]   Tamboli JA, Mohite SK. Development of solid self-microemulsifying drug delivery system of diacerein for enhanced dissolution rate. Asian J Pharm Clin Res 2019; 12(2): 315-9.
[http://dx.doi.org/10.22159/ajpcr.2019.v12i2.29500]

[16] Nanda Kishore R, Yalavarthi PR, Vadlamudi HC, Vandana KR, Rasheed A, Sushma M. Solid self microemulsification of Atorvastatin using hydrophilic carriers: a design. Drug Dev Ind Pharm 2015; 41(7): 1213-22.
[http://dx.doi.org/10.3109/03639045.2014.938655] [PMID: 25019500]

[17] Vadlamudi HC, Yalavarthi PR, M v BR, Rasheed A, N T. *In vitro* characterization studies of self-microemulsified bosentan systems. Drug Dev Ind Pharm 2017; 43(6): 989-95.
[http://dx.doi.org/10.1080/03639045.2017.1287720] [PMID: 28121194]

[18] Silva LAD, Almeida SL, Alonso ECP, *et al.* Preparation of a solid self-microemulsifying drug delivery system by hot-melt extrusion. Int J Pharm 2018; 541(1-2): 1-10.
[http://dx.doi.org/10.1016/j.ijpharm.2018.02.020] [PMID: 29458210]

[19] Balakrishnan P, Lee BJ, Oh DH, *et al.* Enhanced oral bioavailability of dexibuprofen by a novel solid self-emulsifying drug delivery system (SEDDS). Eur J Pharm Biopharm 2009; 72(3): 539-45.
[http://dx.doi.org/10.1016/j.ejpb.2009.03.001] [PMID: 19298857]

[20] Nikolakakis I, Partheniadis I. Self-emulsifying granules and pellets: Composition and formation mechanisms for instant or controlled release. Pharmaceutics 2017; 9(4): 50-62.
[http://dx.doi.org/10.3390/pharmaceutics9040050] [PMID: 29099779]

[21] Seo A, Holm P, Kristensen HG, Schaefer T. The preparation of agglomerates containing solid dispersions of diazepam by melt agglomeration in a high shear mixer. Int J Pharm 2003; 259(1-2): 161-71.
[http://dx.doi.org/10.1016/S0378-5173(03)00228-X] [PMID: 12787644]

[22] Weerapol Y, Limmatvapirat S, Takeuchi H, Sriamornsak P. Fabrication of spontaneous emulsifying powders for improved dissolution of poorly water-soluble drugs. Powder Technol 2015; 271: 100-8.
[http://dx.doi.org/10.1016/j.powtec.2014.10.037]

[23] Gupta S, Kesarla R, Omri A. Formulation strategies to improve the bioavailability of poorly absorbed drugs with special emphasis on self-emulsifying systems. ISRN Pharm 2013; 2013848043
[http://dx.doi.org/10.1155/2013/848043] [PMID: 24459591]

[24] Dokania S, Joshi AK. Self-microemulsifying drug delivery system (SMEDDS)--challenges and road ahead. Drug Deliv 2015; 22(6): 675-90.
[http://dx.doi.org/10.3109/10717544.2014.896058] [PMID: 24670091]

[25] Milind PW, Singh PK, Chaudhari CS, Khairnar DA. Solid self-emulsifying drug delivery system: Preparation techniques and dosage forms. Int J Biopharm 2014; 5(2): 101-8.

[26] https://www.ukessays.com/essays/engineering/advantages-and-disadvantages-of-table-s-in-pharmaceutical-industry engineering-essay.php

[27] Nazzal S, Khan MA. Controlled release of a self-emulsifying formulation from a tablet dosage form: stability assessment and optimization of some processing parameters. Int J Pharm 2006; 315(1-2): 110-21.
[http://dx.doi.org/10.1016/j.ijpharm.2006.02.019] [PMID: 16563673]

[28] Prajapati ST, Patel AN, Patel CN. Formulation and evaluation of controlled-release tablet of zolpidem tartrate by melt granulation technique. ISRN Pharm 2011; 2011208394
[http://dx.doi.org/10.5402/2011/208394] [PMID: 22389845]

[29] Nazzal S, Smalyukh II, Lavrentovich OD, Khan MA. Preparation and *in vitro* characterization of a eutectic based semisolid self-nanoemulsified drug delivery system (SNEDDS) of ubiquinone: mechanism and progress of emulsion formation. Int J Pharm 2002; 235(1-2): 247-65.
[http://dx.doi.org/10.1016/S0378-5173(02)00003-0] [PMID: 11879759]

[30] Chaus HA, Chopade VV, Chaudhri PD. Self-emulsifying drug delivery system: A review. Int J Pharm Chem Sci 2013; 1(2): 34-44.

[31] Bragagni M, Mennini N, Maestrelli F, Cirri M, Mura P. Comparative study of liposomes,

transfersomes and ethosomes as carriers for improving topical delivery of celecoxib. Drug Deliv 2012; 19(7): 354-61.
[http://dx.doi.org/10.3109/10717544.2012.724472] [PMID: 23043648]

[32]   Ito Y, Kusawake T, Ishida M, Tawa R, Shibata N, Takada K. Oral solid gentamicin preparation using emulsifier and adsorbent. J Control Release 2005; 105(1-2): 23-31.
[http://dx.doi.org/10.1016/j.jconrel.2005.03.017] [PMID: 15908031]

[33]   Gala U, Miller D, Williams RO III. Improved dissolution and pharmacokinetics of abiraterone through kinetisol enabled amorphous solid dispersions. Pharmaceutics 2020; 12(4): E357-70.
[http://dx.doi.org/10.3390/pharmaceutics12040357] [PMID: 32295245]

[34]   Agrawal S, Giri TK, Alexander A. A review on novel therapeutic strategies for the enhancement of solubility for hydrophobic drugs through lipid and surfactant based self-microemulsifying drug delivery system: A novel approach. Am J Drug Disc Dev 2012; 2(4): 143-83.
[http://dx.doi.org/10.3923/ajdd.2012.143.183]

[35]   Toorisaka E, Hashida M, Kamiya N, Ono H, Kokazu Y, Goto M. An enteric-coated dry emulsion formulation for oral insulin delivery. J Control Release 2005; 107(1): 91-6.
[http://dx.doi.org/10.1016/j.jconrel.2005.05.022] [PMID: 16039746]

[36]   Bamba J, Cave G, Bensouda Y, Tchoreloff P, Puisieux F, Couarraze G. Cryoprotection of emulsions in freeze-drying: freezing process analysis. Drug Dev Ind Pharm 1995; 21(15): 1749-60.
[http://dx.doi.org/10.3109/03639049509069262]

[37]   Corveleyn S, Remon JP. Formulation of a lyophilized dry emulsion tablet for the delivery of poorly soluble drugs. Int J Pharm 1998; 166(1): 65-74.
[http://dx.doi.org/10.1016/S0378-5173(98)00024-6]

[38]   Myers SL, Shively ML. Preparation and characterization of emulsifiable glasses: Oil-in-water and water-in-oil-in-water emulsions. J Colloid Interface Sci 1992; 149(1): 271-88.
[http://dx.doi.org/10.1016/0021-9797(92)90414-H]

[39]   Patil P, Paradkar A. Porous polystyrene beads as carriers for self-emulsifying system containing loratadine. AAPS PharmSciTech 2006; 7(1): E199-205.
[http://dx.doi.org/10.1208/pt070128] [PMID: 28290043]

[40]   Franceschinis E, Bortoletto C, Perissutti B, Zotto MD, Voinovich D. Self-emulsifying pellets in a lab-scale high shear mixer: Formulation and production design. Powder Technol 2011; 207: 113-8.
[http://dx.doi.org/10.1016/j.powtec.2010.10.016]

[41]   Wang Z, Sun J, Wang Y, *et al.* Solid self-emulsifying nitrendipine pellets: preparation and *in vitro/in vivo* evaluation. Int J Pharm 2010; 383(1-2): 1-6.
[http://dx.doi.org/10.1016/j.ijpharm.2009.08.014] [PMID: 19698771]

[42]   Ingle LM, Wankhade VP, Udasi TA, Tapar KK. New approaches for development and characterization of SMEDDS. Int J Pharm Sci Res 2013; 3(1): 7-14.

[43]   Allen LV. J Pharm Care Pain Symptom Control 2010; 1: 17-26.
[http://dx.doi.org/10.1300/J088v05n02_03]

[44]   Shah I. 2011.

[45]   Dahiya M, Saha S, Shahiwala AF. A review on mouth dissolving films. Curr Drug Deliv 2009; 6(5): 469-76.
[http://dx.doi.org/10.2174/156720109789941713] [PMID: 19751197]

[46]   Xiao L, Yi T, Liu Y, Zhou H. The *in vitro* lipolysis of lipid-based drug delivery systems: A newly identified relationship between drug release and liquid crystalline phase. BioMed Res Int 2016; 20162364317
[http://dx.doi.org/10.1155/2016/2364317] [PMID: 27294110]

[47]   Dixit M, Kulkarni P, Sojan J, *et al.* Formulation and evaluation of positively charged self-emulsifying

drug delivery system containing a NSAID. Int J Pharma Sci 2011; 2(3): 792-03.

[48]   Chen Y, Chen C, Zheng J, Chen Z, Shi Q, Liu H. Development of a solid supersaturatable self-emulsifying drug delivery system of docetaxel with improved dissolution and bioavailability. Biol Pharm Bull 2011; 34(2): 278-86.
[http://dx.doi.org/10.1248/bpb.34.278] [PMID: 21415541]

[49]   Gao P, Morozowich W, Morozowich W. Development of supersaturatable self-emulsifying drug delivery system formulations for improving the oral absorption of poorly soluble drugs. Expert Opin Drug Deliv 2006; 3(1): 97-110.
[http://dx.doi.org/10.1517/17425247.3.1.97] [PMID: 16370943]

[50]   Pandey P, Purohit D, Dureja H. Nanosponges -A promising novel drug delivery system. Recent Pat Nanotechnol 2018; 12(3): 180-91.
[http://dx.doi.org/10.2174/1872210512666180925102842] [PMID: 30251614]

[51]   Chu J, Cheng YL, Rao AV, Nouraei M, Zarate-Muñoz S, Acosta EJ. Lecithin-linker formulations for self-emulsifying delivery of nutraceuticals. Int J Pharm 2014; 471(1-2): 92-102.
[http://dx.doi.org/10.1016/j.ijpharm.2014.05.001] [PMID: 24810240]

[52]   Silpa CR, Krishnakumar K, Smitha KN. Nano sponges: A targeted drug delivery system and its applications 2019.

[53]   Josef E, Bianco-Peled H. Sponges carrying self-microemulsifying drug delivery systems. Int J Pharm 2013; 458(1): 208-17.
[http://dx.doi.org/10.1016/j.ijpharm.2013.09.024] [PMID: 24096300]

[54]   Warke S, Warke P, Kale MK, Saini V. Formulation design and evaluation of herbal self microemulsifying drug delivery system (SMEDDS). Res J Pharm Technol 2011; 4(7): 1135-9.

CHAPTER 8

Herbal Self-emulsifying Formulations

Ravinder Verma[1]**, Deepak Kaushik**[1]**, Vineet Mittal**[1,*] **and Sarita Khatkar**[2]

[1] *Department of Pharmaceutical Sciences, Maharshi Dayanand University, Rohtak (Haryana), 124001, India*

[2] *Vaish Institute of Pharmaceutical Education and Research, Rohtak (Haryana), 124001, India*

Abstract: Herbal drugs have been utilized for a large number of years in the east and ongoing popularity among customers on the planet. These days, 80% of the total populace use pharmaceuticals, which are obtained from plants. Around the world, such drugs make up a 25% of the pharmaceutical armory. SEDDS has a potential for enhancing the bioavailability of inadequately ingested plant parts/actives. Both the crude herb and the extract consist of confounded blends of natural synthetics, which may incorporate unsaturated fats, sterols, alkaloids, flavonoids, glycosides, saponins, tannins and terpenes. Be that as it may, a large portion of herbal constituents are poorly water-soluble and have lipophilic features and reduce distribution, prompting diminished bioavailability and subsequently diminished treatment efficiency, thus requiring repetitive administration or enlarged dose. A variety of herbal drugs and conventional pharmaceuticals being exploited for the formulation of SMEDDS are either extracts or consist of volatile and fixed oils such as zedoary turmeric oil, quercetin, kaempferia parviflora, silymarin, baicalein, hesperidin, curcumin, vinpocetine, nobiletin, oridonin, apigenin, berberine, puerarin and so on which have been discussed here in brief. The nanosized NDDS of herbal drugs has a potential future for upgrading the action and defeating issues related to herbal drugs. This chapter highlights the preformulation study and various phytoconstituents used for the development of SEFs.

Keywords: Bioavailability, Herbal SEFs, Phytoconstituents, Silybin SMEDDS, Vinpocetine, Zedoary turmeric oil.

INTRODUCTION

Some parts of plants, such as leaves, stems, flowers, roots and seeds are usually defined as herbs that have been in use since ancient times and ongoing popularity among customers on the planet. These days, 80% of the total populace consumes pharmaceuticals obtained from plants. Around the world, such drugs make up a 25% of the pharmaceutical armory.

* **Corresponding author Vineet Mittal:** Department of Pharmaceutical Sciences, Maharshi Dayanand University, Rohtak (Haryana), 124001, India; Tel: +91-9812310102; E-mail: vineetmpharma@gmail.com

Herbal drugs are extracted in the form of an extract for which there are various techniques (percolation, maceration, decoction, *etc.*). Percolation is defined as a form of extraction in which the herbs are paced in water, alcohol or different solvents to form an extract that consists of therapeutically active constituents of the plant. Concentrated liquids, pastes or powders are obtained by further warming and drying of these liquid extracts. Both the crude herbs and the extracts consist of confounded blends of natural synthetics, which may incorporate unsaturated fats, sterols, flavonoids, alkaloids, terpenes, saponins, glycosides and tannins. Be that as it may, a large portion of phytoconstituents are poorly water-soluble and have lipophilic features and reduced distribution, prompting diminished bioavailability and subsequently diminished treatment efficiency and need repetitive ingestion or enlarged dose.

In the previous decades, impressive consideration has been centered on the advancement of novel drug delivery systems (NDDS) for herbal drugs. In as of late research, creating nano-sized nanoparticles, nanocapsules, liposomes, SLNs and nanoemulsions have a lot of benefits for herbal drugs in upgrading their bioavailability and solubility, security from toxicity, improvement of therapeutic potential, enrichment of stability, upgrading tissue macrophages distribution, sustained delivery, shielding from chemical and physical degradation. Thus, the nanosized NDDS of herbal drugs has a prospective future for upgrading the therapeutic potential and solving issues related to herbal drugs.

SEDDS has emerged as a potential for enhancing the bioavailability of inadequately ingested plant parts/actives such as mangiferin, tanshinones, patchoulic alcohol and lutin [1].

"SEDDS are defined as an isotropic solution, comprising of oils, surfactants, co-surfactants and drugs which can suddenly create o/w micro/nanoemulsion when blended with the water by mild agitation". It is a wide term, often creating emulsions with a droplet size of nanometers to a few microns. Due to their small size of globules, the micro/nanoemulsified drug can effortlessly be retained through SEDDS. SMEDDS indicates formulations creating clear microemulsion with oil globules in the range of 100-250 nm. SNEDDS is a modern term in which droplet size extends from 50-100 nm [2].

PREFORMULATION INVESTIGATION

When SE herbal formulations interact with the fluids of GI, their fate is quite erratic. The preformulation investigations consider the phase equilibrium investigation and provide a thought regarding the dispersion of SE herbal preparation.

It additionally gives an important assessment about the phase that creates *in vivo* [3]. The magnificence of SMEDDS is self-emulsification which can be changed by the incorporation of phytoconstituents in the preparation. The earlier knowledge regarding the mutual solubility of ingredients is valuable for the development of a transparent, stable and SE formulation [4]. Furthermore, to lessen the possibility of phytoconstituent's precipitation on dispersion, preformulation investigations such as the solvent capacity, *in vitro* digestion and dispersion evaluation must also be carried out one by one for the selected oils [5]. Further, their chemical stability in the formulation is also affected by the presence of the trace contaminants such as peroxide and aldehydes in the lipidic ingredients. Also, the presence of saturated MGs in lipids tends to create haziness in the preparation. So, the manufacturer data sheet should be consulted in brief prior to an assortment of oils [6].

FORMULATION OF SEDDS

The solution of lipid and phytoconstituents are blended with selected surfactants at a specific temperature to produce SE herbal preparation. In preparation, antioxidants such as vitamin E, β-carotene and propyl gallate are incorporated to avoid oxidation. Globule size of oil droplets directly affects the drug discharge rate. The decrease in the molecule size of oil droplets expands the surface milieu of molecules, which gives greater interfacial surface zone and negative interfacial tension. The miniature molecule size of the oil droplets diminishes the thickness of the diffusion layer that results in an upgraded dissolution rate and bioavailability (BA) of plant actives. The distinctive methods like nano milling, HPH and sonication are utilized to build up uniform and stable SE preparations with globule size in nanorange that upgrades the rate of dissolution and hence, the assimilation rate of the drug improved. Further, the preparation with globule size <1000 nm is also predicted to boost solubility, as depicted by Ostwald-Freundlich [7].

SELECTION OF PHYTOCONSTITUENT

These days, the greater part of the analysts trusts that the aqueous solubility of an extract acts as a crucial factor in the development of their SMEDDS preparation. "The Lipinski's rule of 5 directs the scientists to decide solubility of a novel candidate in the aqueous phase." The PWS constituents with a high log P value of 4 (curcumin and limonene) are chiefly developed SEDDS formulation utilizing lipophilic ingredients. But, plant active constituents with inadequate water solubility do not need to be essentially hydrophobic such as oil of vanillin and nutmeg having a log P value of 2. These types of phytoconstituents can be developed as Type IIIB and IV preparation with hydrophilic ingredients or by various methodologies such as nano milling or polymorphism.

In brief, it can be concluded that factors deciding the water solubility are ambiguous to a certain extent due to variation of physicochemical and physiological performance of herbal constituents and therefore, these are required to be evaluated on an individual basis [7].

SELECTION OF INGREDIENTS

It is quite difficult to choose ingredients that are non-toxic and harmless. Commonly, the MCTs are a major alternative as oils in the development of these types of formulations. The selected ingredients should have the greater solvent capability for phytoconstituents and lipophilic surfactant, which is not liable for oxidation. Though, oils can demonstrate distinct physicochemical features or complex toxic interactions with other excipients *in vivo*. Additionally, nanorange cytotoxic components are produced by SNEDDS. Besides this, they are toxic and irritant. It is a chief challenge that need the sensitive tackling during their assortment for specific preparation. Thus, researchers engaged in the development of SMEDDS should consult the USFDA for the selection of ingredients with GRAS status. Furthermore, FDA also keeps up a record of ingredients entitled 'Inactive Ingredient Guide (IIG level)' having the database of ingredients accepted and utilized in commercial products that can be a resource for choosing ingredients [8 - 10].

SEFS FOR PHYTOCONSTITUENTS

A variety of herbal drugs and conventional pharmaceuticals (extracts/volatile oil/fixed oil) are being exploited for SEFs.

Silybin acquired from *Carduus marianus* is evaluated for thriving in shielding cells of the liver from destructive outcomes produced due to alcohol consumption, overworking, smoking, stress, environmental contaminants or drugs that are harmful to the liver. Its chemical structure is depicted in Fig. (**1**). Its low aqueous solubility results in low oral bioavailability. Silybin loaded SMEDDS formulation enhanced about 2.2-folds in comparison with the hard capsule in fasted state dogs [11].

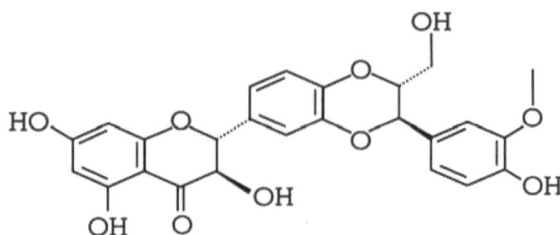

Fig. (1). Chemical structure of silybin.

Dry rhizome is utilized for extraction of zedoary turmeric oil (ZTO) from *Curcuma zedoaria* (Zingiberaceae). ZTO loaded SE microsphere is fabricated with the method of quasi-emulsion-solvent-diffusion for enhancing *in vivo* assimilation. The components of the system were hydroxypropyl methylcellulose acetic acid succinate (HPMCAS-LG), aerosil 200, talc powder and 6.8 phosphate media. The release rate of ZTO from the microsphere was enhanced fundamentally with a greater quantity of dispersing agents and the efficiency of self-emulsification mainly depends on the ratio of HPMCAS-LG and aerosil. The globules of emulsion created from the microsphere have a lesser globule size than SEDDS [13].

Further, a Chinese formulation *Fructus Schisandral Chinensis* developed as SEDDS for enhanced BA and solubility. This plant helps in bringing down the unusual serum glutamic pyruvic transaminase level of patients in the case of acute or chronic hepatitis [14].

Quercetin-loaded microemulsion (containing 0.02: 1:0.2 of lecithin:solutol HS15®:castor) was produced and compared to the pure drug for *in vivo* investigations whose chemical structure is shown in Fig. (**2**). This formulation inhibited the eosinophil enrollment to broncho-alveolar lavage fluid and drastically lessened the level of both IL-5 and IL-4. This also lessened kappa B factor, expression of P-selectin and generation of mucus in lungs. It also displayed the therapeutic potential for inflammation in a murine model [15].

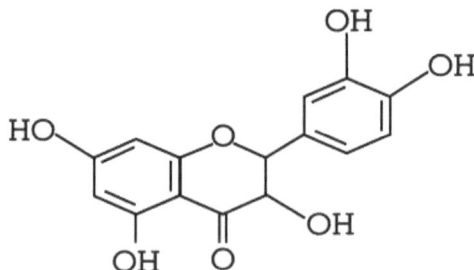

Fig. (2). Chemical structure of quercetin.

Kaempferia parviflora is used as a natural drug for quite a long time in Asia for diverse biological actions. The featured components present in this herb are polymethoxyflavones, as shown in Fig. (3). They belong to BCS class IV. SMEDDS were produced by the use of 53.3% castor oil, 26.7% of propylene glycol and 20% of coconut oil. The oral bioavailability of SMEDDS preparation was superior than its extracts (25.38, 42.00, and 26.01-times for these extracts) [16].

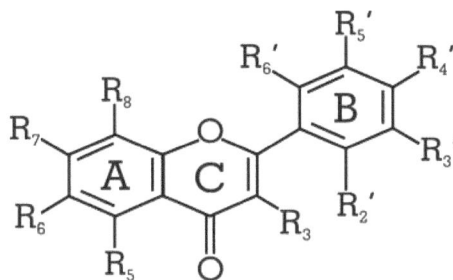

Polymethoxyflavones (PMFs)

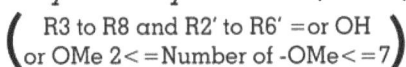

(R3 to R8 and R2′ to R6′ =or OH
or OMe 2<=Number of -OMe<=7)

Fig. (3). Chemical structure of polymethoxyflavones.

In another study, silymarin extract (silybin) loaded SMEDDS that contained ethyl linoleate (10%), cremophor EL (30%) and ethyl alcohol (60%). The bioavailability was extended approximately 2.2-times contrasted with the extract in fasting dogs [17].

Baicalein obtained from the root part of *Scutellaria baicalensis* which has many therapeutic effects but its inadequate aqueous dissolvability is restrictive to its bio-effectiveness. Its chemical structure is demonstrated in Fig. (4). SMEDDS preparation of baicalein consists of 53.57% cremophor RH40, 21.43%t of transcutol P and 25% of caprylic capric acid. The drug discharge rate from SMEDDS was appreciably superior to that of baicalein suspension. *In vivo* investigation demonstrated that its assimilation from SMEDDS increased its relative bioavailability by about 200% compared to baicalein suspension [18].

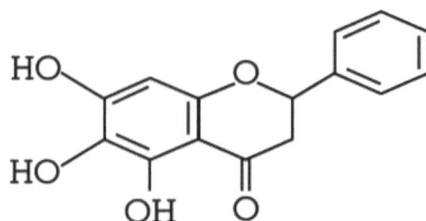

Fig. (4). Chemical structure of baicalein.

The extract of *Rhizoma corydalis* Decumbentis was formulated as SNEDDS utilizing solutol, ethyl oleate and transcutol P as ingredients. SNEDDS demonstrated superior bioavailability as compared to tablets [19].

Hesperidin loaded SMEDDS were produced by using cremophor EL35, isopropyl myristate (IPM) and PEG 400. The globule size of the formulation was found to be less than 100 nm which resulted in enhancement of the assimilation rate of this phytoconstituent [20].

Vinpocetine loaded SMEDDS improved oral bioavailability to almost double (1.91 folds) utilizing labrafac, cremophor EL, oleic acid and transcutol HP. The improved BA might be because of upgrading in discharge, lymphatic transportation and intestinal transfer of drug [21].

Nobiletin loaded SMEDDS were formulated using triethylamine oil, castor oil, polyoxyethylene 35 and tween 80. It was found to have a greater assimilation rate than sub microemulsion and comparable micelles *in vivo*. Furthermore, SMEDDS were more stable than the micelles [22]. Its chemical structure is depicted in Fig. (5).

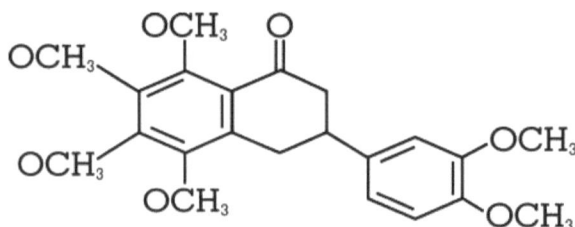

Fig. (5). Chemical structure of nobiletin.

Oridonin loaded SMEDDS were developed using maisine-35, labrafac CC, transcutol P and cremophor EL. The assimilation rate of oridonin from SMEDDS resulted in 2.2 folds upgradation as compared to the suspension form [23].

For enhancing the oral assimilation of silymarin, SMEDDS is considered as a suitable alternative dosage form for this phytoconstituent. They were formulated with tween 80, miglyol and transcutol HP. It was found that the dissolution of silymarin from SMEDDS was superior to marketed formulations [24].

Ginkgo biloba extract loaded SMEDDS were formulated utilizing ethyl oleate, tween 80, 1, 2-propanediol and cremophor EL35. This SMEDDS formulation improved 2.6 folds bioavailability as compared with suspension form [25].

Apigenin loaded SMEDDS consists of kolliphor EL (60%), transcutol P (30%) and capryol 90 (10%). Dissolution investigation illustrated that the drug discharge enhanced approximately 95% from SMEDDS [26].

The berberine hydrochloride loaded SMEDDS was formulated utilizing 40% of ethyl linoleate, 35% of oleic acid, 25% mixture of tween 80 and glycerol. SMEDDS formulation demonstrated high stability and complete drug discharge within 5 hours and C_{max} was considerably improved in comparison to the marketed tablet. SMEDDS formulation improved oral bioavailability to about 2.42 folds than marketed tablet [27]. Its chemical structure is depicted in Fig. (6).

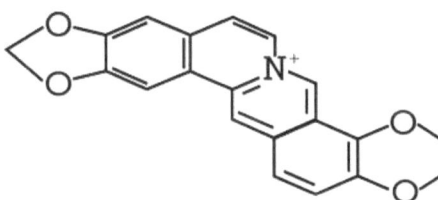

Fig. (6). Chemical structure of berberine.

Puerarin loaded SE sustained-release pellets were formulated by using castor oil, PG and kolliphor EL. The oral BA of SE formulation was improved by 2.6 folds in comparison to the marketed tablet [28].

Hydroxy safflor yellow A loaded self-double emulsifying preparation was formulated by solubilizing PLs in combination with labrafac, tween 80, lipophile WL1349 and oleic acid. This product showed twenty times increment in C_{max} and thirty five times elevation in the AUC value of phytoconstituent in comparison to the aqueous solution of the drug [29].

Gentiopicrin loaded SMEDDS were formulated utilizing phospholipids in kolliphor EL, labrasol and transcutol HP. Gentiopicrin SMEDDS with PLs improved the relative BA of phytoconstituent to about seven times in contrast to extract form.

PLs-complex of morin was formed as SNEDDS utilizing labrafil M1944 CS, kolliphor RH40 and transcutol HP as ingredients which demonstrated a sufficient increment in C_{max}, T_{max} and BA (6.23 times) in comparison to the suspension form of morin [30].

Etoposide loaded phospholipid complex was developed as SEDDS (EPC-SEDDS) with octyl, kolliphor EL, decyl MGs and PEG 400 that improved discharge of drug by 1.21-times and 2.75-times in comparison to its PL complex suspension (EPCS) and simple suspension (ES) form. Apart from this, oral bioavailability of etoposide (ES), EPC-SEDDS and EPCS were improved by 60.21, 44.9 and 8.44 times in comparison to suspension form in animals (rat) [31].

Lutein loaded SNEDDS was formulated with phosal 53, labrosol and transcutol HP. SNEDDS showed rapid dissolution in comparison to marketed product (Eyelac®) but there is no dissolution within a particular time [32]. The enhanced assimilation and bioavailability of phytoconstituents were proposed because of the digestion of PL-drug complex by lipase enzyme into chylomicrons that carries drug atom fundamental assimilation through the lymphatic system.

Some portion of the literature work on Herbal SEFs is shown in Table **1**.

Table 1. The literature work on Herbal SEFs.

Drug	Oil	Surfactant	Co-surfactant/ co-solvent	Type	Carrier	References
Etoposide	Capmul MCM	Polysorbate 80	Transcutol HP	SMEDDS	-	33
Dronedarone	-	Labrafil M 1944CS	Kolliphor EL	SMEDDS		34
PEG-30-dipolyhydroxystearate	Capmul MCM	Cithrol DPHS	Kolliphor HS 15	SMEDDS	-	35
Leuprolein oleate	Capmul MCM (10%)	PG (30%)	Captex 355 (30%)	SMEDDS	-	36
Curcumin	Ethyl oleate (30%)	--	Transcutol HP (17.5%)	Plug tablet	Talcum (1%)	37
Celastrol (10% w/w)	Ethyl oleate (25%)	OP-10 (60%)	Transcutol HP (15%)	SMEDDS		38

Drug	Oil	Surfactant	Co-surfactant/ co-solvent	Type	Carrier	References
Pueraria Flavones	Crodamol GTCC, Maisine 35	Cremophor RH 40	1,2propylene glycol and polyethylene glycol 6000	SMEDDS	-	39
Silmyrin	Ethyl linoleate	Tween 80	Ethyl alcohol	-	-	40
Buparvaquone	Capryol 90 (9.82%)	Kolliphor EL (70.72%)	Labrasol (17.68%)	-	-	41
Paenol and borneol	Ethyl oleate (20%)	Cremophor EL (45%)	Transcutol P (35%)	-	-	42
Mangiferin phospholipid	Cremophor EL 35 (48%)	Labrasol (32%)	-	-	-	43
Paeony glycoside	Ethyl oleate (16.27%)	Cremophor RH 40 (43.34%)	Transcutol P (18.70%)	-	-	44
Dutasteride	Capryol 90 (39.25%)	Cremophor EL (25.90%)	Transcutol HP (34.3%)	-	-	45
25-OCH$_3$-PPD	Labrafil M1944 (30%)	Cremophor EL (50%)	Glycerin (20%)	-	-	46
Oleanic acid	Ethyl oleate(15%)	Cremophor EL (35%)	Ethanol (50%)	-		47
Sirolimus	Labrafil M 1944 CS	Kolliphor EL	Transcutol HP	-	MCC, Na-MCC, lactose	48

CONSENT FOR PUBLICATION

Not applicable.

CONFLICT OF INTEREST

The author declares no conflict of interest, financial or otherwise.

ACKNOWLEDGEMENTS

Declared none.

REFERENCE

[1]   Zhang L, Zhang L, Zhang M, *et al.* Self-emulsifying drug delivery system and the applications in herbal drugs. Drug Deliv 2015; 22(4): 475-86.
        [http://dx.doi.org/10.3109/10717544.2013.861659] [PMID: 24321014]

[2]   Verma R, Kaushik D. Design and optimization of candesartan loaded self-nanoemulsifying drug delivery system for improving its dissolution rate and pharmacodynamic potential 2020.

[3]   Pouton CW. Self-emulsifying drug delivery systems: assessment of the efficiency of emulsification. Int J Pharm 1985; 27(2-3): 335-48.
        [http://dx.doi.org/10.1016/0378-5173(85)90081-X]

[4]   Pouton CW, Porter CJ. Formulation of lipid-based delivery systems for oral administration: materials, methods and strategies. Adv Drug Deliv Rev 2008; 60(6): 625-37.
        [http://dx.doi.org/10.1016/j.addr.2007.10.010] [PMID: 18068260]

[5]   Kaukonen AM, Boyd BJ, Porter CJ, Charman WN. Drug solubilization behavior during *in vitro* digestion of simple triglyceride lipid solution formulations. Pharm Res 2004; 21(2): 245-53.
        [http://dx.doi.org/10.1023/B:PHAM.0000016282.77887.1f] [PMID: 15032305]

[6]   Cao Y, Marra M, Anderson BD. Predictive relationships for the effects of triglyceride ester concentration and water uptake on solubility and partitioning of small molecules into lipid vehicles. J Pharm Sci 2004; 93(11): 2768-79.
        [http://dx.doi.org/10.1002/jps.20126] [PMID: 15389678]

[7]   Chouhan N, Mittal V, Kaushik D, Khatkar A, Raina M. Self emulsifying drug delivery system (SEDDS) for phytoconstituents: a review. Curr Drug Deliv 2015; 12(2): 244-53.
        [http://dx.doi.org/10.2174/1567201811666141021142606] [PMID: 25335929]

[8]   www.fda.gov/Food/IngredientsPackagingLabeling/GRAS/default.htm

[9]   www.accessdata.fda.gov/ scripts/cder/iig/index.cfm

[10]   Brown AC. An overview of herb and dietary supplement efficacy, safety and government regulations in the United States with suggested improvements. Part 1 of 5 series. Food Chem Toxicol 2017; 107(Pt A): 449-71.
        [http://dx.doi.org/10.1016/j.fct.2016.11.001] [PMID: 27818322]

[11]   Di Costanzo A, Angelico R. Formulation strategies for enhancing the bioavailability of silymarin: The state of the art. Molecules 2019; 24(11): 2155-65.
        [http://dx.doi.org/10.3390/molecules24112155] [PMID: 31181687]

[12]   Li X, Yuan Q, Huang Y, Zhou Y, Liu Y. Development of silymarin self-microemulsifying drug delivery system with enhanced oral bioavailability. AAPS PharmSciTech 2010; 11(2): 672-8.
        [http://dx.doi.org/10.1208/s12249-010-9432-x] [PMID: 20405254]

[13]   Zhao Y, Wang C, Chow AH, *et al.* Self-nanoemulsifying drug delivery system (SNEDDS) for oral delivery of Zedoary essential oil: formulation and bioavailability studies. Int J Pharm 2010; 383(1-2): 170-7.
        [http://dx.doi.org/10.1016/j.ijpharm.2009.08.035] [PMID: 19732813]

[14]   Sapra G, Vyas YK, Agarwal R, Aggarwal A, Chandrashekar KT, Sharma K. Effect of an herb root extract, herbal dentifrice and synthetic dentifrice on human salivary amylase. Dent Res J (Isfahan) 2013; 10(4): 493-8.
        [PMID: 24130585]

[15]   Rogerio AP, Dora CL, Andrade EL, *et al.* Anti-inflammatory effect of quercetin-loaded microemulsion in the airways allergic inflammatory model in mice. Pharmacol Res 2010; 61(4): 288-97.
        [http://dx.doi.org/10.1016/j.phrs.2009.10.005] [PMID: 19892018]

[16]   Mekjaruskul C, Yang YT, Leed MG, Sadgrove MP, Jay M, Sripanidkulchai B. Novel formulation

strategies for enhancing oral delivery of methoxyflavones in *Kaempferia parviflora* by SMEDDS or complexation with 2-hydroxypropyl-β-cyclodextrin. Int J Pharm 2013; 445(1-2): 1-11.
[http://dx.doi.org/10.1016/j.ijpharm.2013.01.052] [PMID: 23376503]

[17]   Wei L, Li G, Yan YD, Pradhan R, Kim JO, Quan Q. Lipid emulsion as a drug delivery system for breviscapine: formulation development and optimization. Arch Pharm Res 2012; 35(6): 1037-43.
[http://dx.doi.org/10.1007/s12272-012-0611-z] [PMID: 22870813]

[18]   Liu W, Tian R, Hu W, *et al.* Preparation and evaluation of self-microemulsifying drug delivery system of baicalein. Fitoterapia 2012; 83(8): 1532-9.
[http://dx.doi.org/10.1016/j.fitote.2012.08.021] [PMID: 22982454]

[19]   Ma H, Zhao Q, Wang Y, Guo T, An Y, Shi G. Design and evaluation of self-emulsifying drug delivery systems of Rhizoma corydalis decumbentis extracts. Drug Dev Ind Pharm 2012; 38(10): 1200-6.
[http://dx.doi.org/10.3109/03639045.2011.643897] [PMID: 22512784]

[20]   Xiaoyan F, Jun L, Wen W. Study on the absorption kinetics of hesperidin self-microemulsion in rat's intestine. Acta Universitatis Medicinalis Anhui 2011; 8: 222-32.

[21]   Chen Y, Li G, Wu X, *et al.* Self-microemulsifying drug delivery system (SMEDDS) of vinpocetine: formulation development and *in vivo* assessment. Biol Pharm Bull 2008; 31(1): 118-25.
[http://dx.doi.org/10.1248/bpb.31.118] [PMID: 18175953]

[22]   Yao J, Lu Y, Zhou JP. Preparation of nobiletin in self-microemulsifying systems and its intestinal permeability in rats. J Pharm Pharm Sci 2008; 11(3): 22-9.
[http://dx.doi.org/10.18433/J3MS3M] [PMID: 18801304]

[23]   Liu Y, Zhang P, Feng N, Zhang X, Wu S, Zhao J. Optimization and in situ intestinal absorption of self-microemulsifying drug delivery system of oridonin. Int J Pharm 2009; 365(1-2): 136-42.
[http://dx.doi.org/10.1016/j.ijpharm.2008.08.009] [PMID: 18782611]

[24]   Liu L, Pang X, Zhang W, Wang S. Formulation design and *in vitro* evaluation of silymarin-loaded self-microemulsifying drug delivery systems. Asian J Pharm Sci 2007; 2(4): 150-60.

[25]   Tang J, Sun J, Cui F, Zhang T, Liu X, He Z. Self-emulsifying drug delivery systems for improving oral absorption of ginkgo biloba extracts. Drug Deliv 2008; 15(8): 477-84.
[http://dx.doi.org/10.1080/10717540802039089] [PMID: 18720135]

[26]   Zhao L, Zhang L, Meng L, Wang J, Zhai G. Design and evaluation of a self-microemulsifying drug delivery system for apigenin. Drug Dev Ind Pharm 2013; 39(5): 662-9.
[http://dx.doi.org/10.3109/03639045.2012.687378] [PMID: 22607130]

[27]   Zhu JX, Tang D, Feng L, *et al.* Development of self-microemulsifying drug delivery system for oral bioavailability enhancement of berberine hydrochloride. Drug Dev Ind Pharm 2013; 39(3): 499-506.
[http://dx.doi.org/10.3109/03639045.2012.683875] [PMID: 22563917]

[28]   Zhang Y, Wang R, Wu J, Shen Q. Characterization and evaluation of self-microemulsifying sustained-release pellet formulation of puerarin for oral delivery. Int J Pharm 2012; 427(2): 337-44.
[http://dx.doi.org/10.1016/j.ijpharm.2012.02.013] [PMID: 22366381]

[29]   Lv LZ, Tong CQ. LV Q, Tang XJ, Li LM, Fang QX, Yu J, Han M, Gao JQ. Enhanced absorption of hydroxysafflor yellow A using a self-double-emulsifying drug delivery system. Int J Nanomedicine 2012; 7: 4099-07.
[PMID: 22888246]

[30]   Schick MJ. Nonionic Surfactants. 1st ed., New York: Marcel Dekker 1977.

[31]   Cui SX, Nie SF, Li L, Wang CG, Pan WS, Sun JP. Preparation and evaluation of self-microemulsifying drug delivery system containing vinpocetine. Drug Dev Ind Pharm 2009; 35(5): 603-11.
[http://dx.doi.org/10.1080/03639040802488089] [PMID: 19040178]

[32]   Yoo JH, Shanmugam S, Thapa P, *et al.* Novel self-nanoemulsifying drug delivery system for enhanced

solubility and dissolution of lutein. Arch Pharm Res 2010; 33(3): 417-26.
[http://dx.doi.org/10.1007/s12272-010-0311-5] [PMID: 20361307]

[33]   Zhao G, Huang J, Xue K, Si L, Li G. Enhanced intestinal absorption of etoposide by self-microemulsifying drug delivery systems: roles of P-glycoprotein and cytochrome P450 3A inhibition. Eur J Pharm Sci 2013; 50(3-4): 429-39.
[http://dx.doi.org/10.1016/j.ejps.2013.08.016] [PMID: 23981337]

[34]   Han SD, Jung SW, Jang SW, Son M, Kim BM, Kang MJ. Reduced foodeffect on intestinal absorption of dronedarone by selfmicroemulsifying drug delivery system. Biol Pharm Bull 2015; 38(7): 1026-32.
[http://dx.doi.org/10.1248/bpb.b15-00110] [PMID: 26133712]

[35]   Tamer H. Hassan, Handrik M, Karsten M. Novel semisolid SNEDDS on PEG-3--dipolyhydroxystearate: Development and characterization. Int J Pharm 2014; 477: 506-18.
[http://dx.doi.org/10.1016/j.ijpharm.2014.10.063] [PMID: 25445530]

[36]   Hintzen F, Perera G, Hauptstein S, Mller C. affleur F, BernkopSchnrch A. *In vivo* evaluation of *in vivo* of an oral SMEDDS for leuprorelin. Int J Pharm 2014; 472(12): 2026.

[37]   Huang Y, Tian R, Hu W, *et al.* A novel plug-controlled colon-specific pulsatile capsule with tablet of curcumin-loaded SMEDDS. Carbohydr Polym 2013; 92(2): 2218-23.
[http://dx.doi.org/10.1016/j.carbpol.2012.11.105] [PMID: 23399280]

[38]   Qi X, Qin J, Ma N, Chou X, Wu Z. Solid self-microemulsifying dispersible tablets of celastrol: formulation development, charaterization and bioavailability evaluation. Int J Pharm 2014; 472(1-2): 40-7.
[http://dx.doi.org/10.1016/j.ijpharm.2014.06.019] [PMID: 24929011]

[39]   Guan Q, Zhang G, Sun S, Fan H, Sun C, Zhang S. Enhanced oral bioavailability of pueraria flavones by a novel solid self-microemulsifying drug delivery system (SMEDDS) dropping pills. Biol Pharm Bull 2016; 39(5): 762-9.
[http://dx.doi.org/10.1248/bpb.b15-00854] [PMID: 26935150]

[40]   Jakki R, Afzal SM, Kandai P, Veerabrahma K. Development of SMEDDS of domperidone: *In vitro* and *in vivo* evaluation. Acta Pharm 2013; 63(2): 241-51.
[http://dx.doi.org/10.2478/acph-2013-0013] [PMID: 23846146]

[41]   Venkatesh G, Majid MI, Mansor SM, Nair NK, Croft SL, Navaratnam V. *In vitro* and *in vivo* evaluation of self-microemulsifying drug delivery system of buparvaquone. Drug Dev Ind Pharm 2010; 36(6): 735-45.
[http://dx.doi.org/10.3109/03639040903460446] [PMID: 20136493]

[42]   Lü FQ, Li H, Xu W, *et al.* [Preparation of self-microemulsion drug delivery system of the mixture of paeonol and borneol based on Xingbi Fang]. Yao Xue Xue Bao 2013; 48(10): 1602-10.
[PMID: 24417089]

[43]   Xuan XY, Wang YJ, Tian H, Pi JX, Sun SZ, Zhang WL. [Study on prescription of self-microemulsifying drug delivery system of mangiferin phospholipid complex]. Zhong Yao Cai 2012; 35(9): 1508-11.
[PMID: 23451508]

[44]   Chen LJ, Liu Y, Liu Y, Li L, Gao F. Enhanced bioavailability of total paeony glycoside by self-microemulsifying drug delivery system. Yao Xue Xue Bao 2012; 47(12): 1678-86.
[PMID: 23460976]

[45]   Choo GH, Park SJ, Hwang SJ, Kim MS. Formulation and *in vivo* evaluation of a self-microemulsifying drug delivery system of dutasteride. Drug Res (Stuttg) 2013; 63(4): 203-9.
[http://dx.doi.org/10.1055/s-0033-1334965] [PMID: 23487399]

[46]   Sermkaew N, Ketjinda W, Boonme P, Phadoongsombut N, Wiwattanapatapee R. Liquid and solid self-microemulsifying drug delivery systems for improving the oral bioavailability of andrographolide from a crude extract of Andrographis paniculata. Eur J Pharm Sci 2013; 50(3-4): 459-66.

[http://dx.doi.org/10.1016/j.ejps.2013.08.006] [PMID: 23973887]

[47]   Yang R, Huang X, Dou J, Zhai G, Su L. Self-microemulsifying drug delivery system for improved oral bioavailability of oleanolic acid: design and evaluation. Int J Nanomedicine 2013; 8: 2917-26. [PMID: 23966781]

[48]   Hu X, Lin C, Chen D, *et al.* Sirolimus solid self-microemulsifying pellets: formulation development, characterization and bioavailability evaluation. Int J Pharm 2012; 438(1-2): 123-33. [http://dx.doi.org/10.1016/j.ijpharm.2012.07.055] [PMID: 22850296]

CHAPTER 9

In Vitro Digestion Models and Pharmacokinetic Aspects of SMEDDS

Deepak Kaushik[1,*] and **Ravinder Verma**[1]

[1] *Department of Pharmaceutical Sciences, Maharshi Dayanand University, Rohtak (Haryana), 124001, India*

Abstract: *In vitro* models evaluate lipid-based drug delivery systems for enhancing solubilization and discharge of the drug. After ingestion, the food particles experience different physical and chemical changes that prompt their fragmentation into little pieces and change into less complex atomic groups that can be effortlessly absorbed into the blood. The dynamic mono and multi-compartmental models have become more advanced with *in vivo* information input. The Dynamic Gastric Model (DGM) has two sections: One is the body and the other is the antrum of the gastric. Up until now, TNO gastro-Intestinal Model-1(TIM-1) is considered to mimic the closest reproduction of the energy and flow of human retention. Pancreatic lipase, bile salts, phospholipids and calcium ions are involved in the intestinal lipolysis. The intestinal lipolysis is typically assessed by the rate and degree of free unsaturated fats discharged due to the activity of P-LIP. These can be estimated utilizing diverse strategies such as colorimetric enzymatic test, gas chromatography and pH-stat titration. The various *in vivo* pharmacokinetic aspects of LBFs are formulation and solubilization, dispersibility, dilution and effect on pharmacokinetics that have been described in this chapter. Other pharmacokinetic parameters including assimilation and bioavailability improvement, the impact of excipient choice on bioavailability, lymphatic transport and food effect reduction have been summarized. This chapter highlights the various *in vitro* digestion models and pharmacokinetic aspects of LBFs.

Keywords: Food effect, *In vitro* digestion models, Intestinal lipolysis, Lymphatic uptake, pH-stat titration, Pharmacokinetic aspects.

DIFFICULTIES, APPROACHES AND LIMITATIONS IN CREATING *IN VITRO* DIGESTION MODELS

As of late, the *in vitro* lipolysis show has given an incredible renovation of the *in vivo* lipid assimilation process. These *in vitro* models are used to evaluate lipid-

* **Corresponding author Deepak Kaushik:** Department of Pharmaceutical Sciences, Maharshi Dayanand University, Rohtak (Haryana), 124001, India; Tel: +91 9315809626; E-mail: deepkaushik1977@gmail.com

based delivery systems for enhancing drug solubilization and discharge rate. Ultracentrifugation can be utilized for the isolation of distinctive lipolysis assimilation phases. The aqueous phase is essential for assimilation, because it colloidal phases and drug break up in the liquid phase is essential for assimilation. The grouping of drug in the watery phase has incredible importance for retention. The sediment phase consists of calcium soaps of unsaturated fats and precipitated drug. It is concluded that the quantity of solid, precipitated drug and the dissolution rate have an impact on retention [1].

Gastrointestinal retention is, to a great degree, intricate and extremely hard to display. After ingestion, the food particles experience different physical and chemical changes that prompt its debasement into the little pieces and change into less complex atomic groups that can be effortlessly exchanged through the absorptive cells. Subsequently, amid displaying assimilation *in vitro*, it is important to the model physiologically [2].

Successful demonstration of human retention is additionally tested by the individual variation in physiological conditions that may rely upon the wellbeing and physical status of the person. The nourishment particles animate the human GIT in various ways.

For instance, there are contrasts in the retention of food proteins relying upon their preparation history such as crude or prepared. Also, ingestion of nourishment rich in proteins, sugars or fats, separately, builds the relative measures of proteases, amylases or lipases in the pancreatic secretion. Another factor is the transit time of each phase, whether it is the stomach or the intestine. Transit time changes from supper to dinner contingent upon the kind of nourishment (type and physical state) which influences its absorbability and ingestion of its segments such as hydrophobic bioactive mixes have constrained assimilation and in this manner, low bioavailability when they have a short upper intestinal travel time. When high-fat substances enter into the gastrointestinal tract, the stomach purging is backed off, thus expanding the travel phase time. Subsequently, these progressions ought to be taken in thought amid demonstrating human digestion [3].

Notwithstanding the progressions in microstructure and physical properties of nourishments amid digestion, the ingestion and bioavailability of the embodied bioactive mixes can likewise be researched *in vitro*, to better outline the practical food systems. Researchers and pharmacologists routinely utilize caco-2 cell lines as a piece of *in vitro* to demonstrate bioavailability affected by food. These cells duplicate *in vitro* the retention and the exchange capacity of intestinal epithelial covering. After *in vitro* lipolysis, the amount of the lipophilic drug that is exchanged through the layer of the covering cells is evaluated and compared with that present inside the cells.

Through years of relevant research, *in vitro* assimilation has been drawn closer in different routes, contingent upon the reason for examination. A significant number of the created models are monocompartmental models that pay attention to a solitary phase of assimilation, regardless of whether it is in the stomach, upper intestine, or lower intestine (normally for microbial greenery ponders). These models are particularly vital as screening devices since they are shoddy, reproducible and utilized with a substantial number of tests. These models do not have the flow and the multifaceted nature of human digestion such as the progressions of pH after some time, stomach emptying and assimilation of retention time [2].

The dynamic mono and multi-compartmental models are more advanced with *in vivo* information input such as the Dynamic Gastric Model (DGM) has two sections - body and the antrum of the gastric. The DGM reproduces gastric purging, utilizing a viscosity valve that allows the entry of little particles first while the bigger parts are sent back to the antrum for shear and crushing [4]. Another case is the TNO gastro-Intestinal Model-1(TIM-1) which is considered, up until now, the closest reproduction of the energy and flow of human retention. Through PC control, it consolidates the key variables of assimilation such as temperature, pH changes, stomach and upper digestive tract exhausting, peristaltic movements, consecutive compound discharge and expulsion of retention items and water through dialysis and filtration systems [2].

In spite of the considerable number of endeavors and the accomplishments in developing the most physiologically relevant *in vitro* digestion model, these systems still miss the mark concerning duplicating certain variables, for example, the part of hormones, apprehensive control and input systems, lining mucosal layers and neighborhood invulnerability [2]. Nonetheless, there exists a requirement for other options for the creature and human examinations. *In vitro* models can help diminish the quantity of concentrates required to be done on living creatures, which is imperative from the exploration morals perspective. They are likewise viable and non-costly regarding assessing the expansive number of nourishment in less time. It is substantially less demanding to gather tests for examining physical, synthetic and microstructure changes in the nourishment systems utilizing the *in vitro*, which takes into account the components to be assessed. However, it is highly important to relate the *in vitro* information with the results obtained from human and creature models [5].

Intestinal Lipolysis

In food items, lipids are the most part in emulsion shape either as the last item or incorporated into a more advanced structure. Lipids increase the value of nourishment through surface, flavor and mouthfeel. Beginning at rumination, the breakdown of the structure causes the arrival of flavor and influences the tangible view of the nourishment particles.

Different lipophilic bioactives are stacked in embodiment emulsion systems and afterwards, brought into nourishment items, *e.g.*, omega-3 unsaturated fats, carotenoids, phytosterols and oil-soluble vitamins.

Be that as it may, there are challenges amid its application because such mixes have low water-dissolvability. They are regularly synthetically temperamental and inadequately bioavailable in the ingestion.

Pancreatic lipase (P-LIP) is an exocrine protein that is responsible for lipid digestion in the duodenum. P-LIP hydrolyzes triacylglycerol particles at sn-2 position into one monoacylglycerol atom and two unsaturated fats. The digestion results are amphiphilic and tend to go to the oil droplet interface. Since lipid retention occurs at the oil-water interface, the collection can anticipate the advanced movement of lipase. The presence of bio-surfactants like bile salts (BS) and polar phospholipids (PLs) potentiate the movement of lipase.

Bile salts help in the clearance of the interface from lipolysis and result in solubilizing and framing blended micelles. Furthermore, they assume a noteworthy part in emulsifying ingested lipids at the low shear powers in the upper digestive tract. The presence of the phospholipids in the medium potentiates the emulsifying impact of bile salts by bringing down interfacial pressure along these lines expanding the aggregate droplet surface zone prepared for retention.

Bile is consistently discharged in the duodenum. It varies from 3-7 mM in the fasting state to 13-46 mM after the postprandial, exhausting of the gall bladder. This extensive increment in the bile focuses on the duodenum bit by bit and declines to just 2.5-10 mM, 30 minutes after dinner. Since bile salts have higher surface activity than lipolysis, they tend to aggregate at the interface and dislodge other surface dynamic atoms. The presence of the co-lipase, a co-factor protein, helps in the adsorption of P-LIP at the interface. Co-lipase and P-LIP shape a coupling complex, while at the same time co-lipase conjugates to the bile salts. It was discovered that co-lipase molecules could go about as micellization cores for bile salts. The association between co-lipase, PLIP and bile salts at the interface encourage the P-LIP to access the interface better and upgrade lipolysis [6].

The presence of phospholipids amid assimilation is likewise exceptionally basic to lipolysis and the exchange of unsaturated fats into blended micelles. All things considered, grown-up people usually consume around 4-8 g of phospholipids everyday, with phosphatidyl choline (PC) as the prevailing sort. Gastric and intestinal phospholipids go about as emulsifiers amid retention of the ingested lipids. In the intestinal lumen, there are roughly 8 g of PC blended with a toll. However, the aggregate phospholipids focus in the duodenum is an exceeding factor and ranges from 0.3-5.5 mM, dependending upon consuming fewer calories and managed by biliary secretion. It was discovered that the phospholipids/bile salts proportion in biliary fistula rats, observed by imbuing taurocholate salts in cannulated bile channels, begins around 0.08-0.014:100 and achieves 6:100 before the finishing of the mixture and that the intra-canaliculi centralization of bile salts emphatically directs the phospholipids secretion. A proportion of 1:4 (phospholipids:bile salts) has been accounted for human stomach related juices. At the point when phospholipids are broken up in water, they frame "huge lamellar structures" that may not be promptly accessible to phospholipases in presence of the bile salts, and phospholipids shape little blended micelles that can be hydrolyzed. Utilizing gastric and intestinal phospholipids in mimicking digestion *in vitro* is dependably a decision of the analysts. It is generally training in non-dynamic *in vitro* models.

Phospholipases are isolated into five gatherings of catalysts relying upon their cleavage activity on various phospholipids. Phospholipase A2 (PLA2) is the most portrayed and examined aggregate among different phospholipases. PLA2 extracted from pancreatic juices is delegated a subdivision of PLA2 gathering that is known as little sub-atomic mass emitted PLA2 (sPLA2) [7]. They are utilized as a part of *in vitro* retention models to hydrolyze phospholipids and copy the physiological enzymatic profile of pancreatic lipases.

Late examinations demonstrated that the expansion of PLA2 and co-lipase into *in vitro* models expands the action of lipases and the micellization of bioactive-typified emulsions amid mimicked intestinal assimilation. Regularly, PLA2 is discharged in the exocrine pancreatic squeezes in a non-dynamic shape, which is then initiated within the presence of trypsin, a pancreatic chemical. It hydrolyzes the glycerol spine at position two and its movement is fundamentally subject to calcium particles as a co-factor.

Another critical factor in intestinal lipolysis is the part that calcium plays in the action of P-LIP. Calcium particles accelerate long-chain free unsaturated fats (LCFA) formed as a result of lipolysis in insoluble cleansers. Along these lines, calcium clears the droplet to the interface for encouraging lipase availability, particularly after bile salt micelles turn out to be excessively immersed with lipolysis side-effects. Calcium has likewise been accounted for starting lipase action without the nearness of co-lipase and bile salts. It goes about as a co-factor that expands the turnover number and decreases the slack period of the P-LIP catalyst. Calcium is additionally a vital factor influencing the movement of other stomach related proteins, for instance, to settle the atomic arrangement of trypsinogen and chymotrypsinogen. To consider the part of calcium in intestinal lipolysis, Hu and collaborators included a sustenance review calcium restricting operator, ethylene di-amine tetra-acidic acid (EDTA) to *in vitro* retention medium. The digestion rate and degree were drastically brought down. The impact was expected to a limited extent to calcium chelation, yet additionally to the inhibitory impact of EDTA and the chelation of other fundamental particles required for lipase movement.

The most normally utilized conveyance systems in nourishment are emulsions. There are a few methodologies for their formulations. These conveyance systems differ in relying on their motivation and capacity. The assessment of intestinal lipolysis of oil in water emulsions utilizing as a part of *in vitro* assimilation models helped better understanding the progressions occurring in their microstructure amid retention. Factors such as droplet size, type of oil, kind of emulsifier, polysaccharide, proteins or other macromolecular structures at the interface have been assessed.

The impact of the presence of both pectin and chitosan in a corn oil/water emulsion-fiber blend on the microstructural during assimilation was examined utilizing *in vitro* digestion. It was discovered that pectin advances exhaustion flocculation of oil droplets at specific concentrations and pH, while chitosan incites crossing over flocculation. Such flocculation keeps the entrance of P-LIP protein and the co-lipase into the interface, which this way diminishes the last degree of lipid retention. These outcomes were affirmed by another investigation in which oil droplets were covered with chitosan and this polymer caused a lessening in the lipid retention rate. Notwithstanding, such discoveries are still under level-headed discussion. Different analysts found no inhibitory impact of chitosan on lipase, as the chitosan edifices desorb from the interface amid assimilation making the interface available to stomach related compounds.

The rate of retention improves with diminishing oil droplet size. The kind of oil likewise influences the energy of assimilation, with quicker retention with the presence of MCT *versus* LCT. The type of emulsifier could also influence the lipase openness to the oil droplet interface. Mun *et al.,* contemplated the *in vitro* assimilation of corn oil/water emulsion utilizing distinctive types of emulsifiers. They found that Tween 20 was the safest, while caseinate and whey protein was the minimum safe [8].

Multilayers could likewise be outlined at the interface of oil droplets, helping in the assurance and the conveyance of practical bioactive mixes.

A few *in vitro* assimilation models have been produced to imitate human digestion and help in assessing the conduct of different nourishments, drugs and ecological poisons amid retention. The intestinal lipolysis is typically assessed by the rate and degree of free unsaturated fats discharge by the activity of P-LIP. The FFA discharged can be estimated utilizing diverse strategies.

For instance, Shimizu *et al.,* estimated FFAs by an enzymatic test that can be utilized as a part of a colorimetric enzymatic NEFA pack for assessing FFA in blood sera. This strategy has been utilized to decide the FFA discharge after *in vitro* retention of o/w emulsion tests [9].

Another approach is using gas chromatography (GC) or different types of chromatography such as thin-layer chromatography and high-pressure liquid chromatography (HPLC). These strategies are considered of high affectability and specificity; however, they are tedious and not nonstop. Specifically, chromatography expedites more itemized data of the lipolysis profile, for instance, lipolysis results arrangement after some time, the chain length of discharged unsaturated fats and their immersion level.

IN VITRO EVALUATION OF LIPID ASSIMILATION

The pH-stat titrimetry method is generally used to assess *in vitro* intestinal lipolysis. Although all the more as of late it has been utilized additionally to repeat *in vitro* the dynamic changes of pH in the stomach amid retention. The pH-stat titrator is a PC mechanized gadget associated with working of the programming. The temperature-controlled retention vessel of the pH-stat can repeat the intestinal conditions (human body temperature at 37°C, duodenal pH 6.5-7.5 and reenacted assimilation of liquid. The titrator has a computerized pH terminal that distinguishes changes in pH because of discharge of the free fatty acid (FFA) amid the assimilation of triacyl glyceride (TAG). It is assumed that the pancreatic lipase hydrolysis yields from each TAG atom to 2 FFAs and one monoacylglycerol. Thus the measure of NaOH consumed is identified with the degree of lipolysis. The pH terminal and the programmed burette has three primary functions: to start with lipase, screen and maintain the pH in human physiology, secondly, keeping up the activity of the pancreatic lipase by keeping the pH-controlled and thirdly, keeping a record of pH changes and NaOH consumed determines the rate and degree of assimilation. The pH-stat strategy is thought to be inside one μmole of discharged is equivalent to unsaturated fat. The synthesis of small intestinal fluid (SIF) is primarily a blend of pancreatic lipase, BS and minerals, including calcium and its concentrations differ while the assimilation in the fed or fasting condition [3].

The distinctive investigations utilizing the pH-stat *in vitro* study demonstrated that the intestinal lipolysis of o/w emulsions contrasts, relying upon the various variables. These variables are intrinsic, *i.e.*, identified with the synthesis of the SIF picked or extraneous, and also with the organization and the outline of the emulsion itself. These elements include oil droplet size, lipid emulsification, pH of titration, calcium ions, SIF development (fundamentally proteins and bile) and the type of emulsifier.

Because of the significance of calcium for the movement of the pancreatic lipase and lipolysis, calcium ions in the SIF are focal points. Usually, the amount of calcium ions in the duodenum amid retention relies upon the eating routine and the measure of calcium present in the nourishment. Calcium bioavailability additionally relies upon the presence of some calcium restricting operators which could be of a natural starting point such as mucin and some inherent proteins or other restricting carriers found in the ingested nourishment. For example, EDTA, phosphates and biopolymers make calcium less accessible for assimilation. Also, calcium is secreted by the pancreatic acinar cells and other pancreatic compounds because of the arrival of the hormones (secretin and cholecystokinin).

The two hormones are secreted by the duodenal epithelium in the presence of the acidic chyme in the duodenum. Another wellspring of calcium in the duodenum is the gall bladder bile juice which contains up to 11 mM of calcium.

Two investigations have been looked at calcium ions concentartion amid digestion and their impact on the rate and degree of lipolysis utilizing calcium at 5, 10 and 20 mM amid *in vitro* retention of emulsions checked at various types of emulsifiers. It was found that higher concentrations of calcium result in the increment of the digestion rate.

Similar outcomes were found by Zangenberg and colleagues (2001) after an investigation on the disintegration of lipophilic drug substances utilizing *in vitro* lipolysis model [10]. Biopolymers like alginate that ties emphatically to the calcium particles, cause a reduction in the rate of assimilation. The effect of calcium and its concentration on the rate of *in vitro* lipolysis was additionally assessed utilizing various types of fats: SCT, MCT or LCT. Calcium was found to affect expanding lipolysis of LCT with MCT and SCT. Although MacGregor and associates (1997) announced that the impact of calcium on *in vitro* lipolysis of SCT is unimportant.

The method of calcium ions increment amid *in vitro* intestinal lipolysis was additionally explored. Incorporating calcium consistently amid *in vitro* retention controls the rate of lipolysis, while the underlying expansion of a higher concentration of calcium expands the rate of lipolysis in the underlying phases of assimilation.

The constant addition favored this technique because of the part of calcium accumulating on long-chain unsaturated fats (LCFA) into surfactants. These LCFA gather at the oil droplet interface and would diminish the rate of lipolysis. Notwithstanding, including calcium consistently amid retention, may not be physiologically applicable, as it might be unique to what is occurring *in vivo*. This is a subject of much open deliberation. Larsen and colleagues (2011) exhibited that utilizing calcium through nonstop addition is valuable to mimic *in vivo* ingestion of FFA. Different strategies used to copy assimilation and expulsion of digestion items; for example, bio-films and dialysis are turned out to be intricate [6]. To additionally consider the part of calcium in the energy of intestinal lipolysis, different researchers utilized distinctive kinds of calcium salts and found that salts of water-soluble calcium such as calcium gluconate, calcium acetic acid derivatives and calcium chloride strongly affect expanding the rate and degree of retention in contrast with the other salts of calcium like calcium oxide or calcium sulphate which are less water-soluble [10].

The activity of pancreatic lipase is ideal between pH 6.5 and 8.0 and the pH of titration for the pH-stat *in vitro* intestinal lipolysis is kept up near unbiased.

Oleic acid, a LCFA, has a clear pKa value around 7.7 and it is non-ionized amid normal pH-stat estimations. The non-ionized FFA particles hasten and result in the underestimation of the aggregate FFA discharged. As it may, past work found that the pKa estimation of the LCFA diminishes when calcium and bile salts are in the medium. Thus, it has been proposed that a "trade-off pH" ought to be picked in the vicinity of 6.5 and 8.5 [11], suggesting a purported "back titration" advance to be directed towards the finish of the pH-stat retention. The pH is raised to 9 (to cover the pKa scope of LCFAs) and the titration is led when all the FFA in the medium are ionized and can be titrated [12].

Role of Chemicals

The most ordinarily utilized lipase for *in vitro* intestinal lipolysis models is pancreatin, a porcine pancreas extract (PPE) containing the principle pancreatic stomach related chemicals. It is expected not exclusively to constrain the business accessibility of human pancreatic lipase (HPL) and co-lipase yet in addition to that way, this blend of chemicals contains extra lipolytic compounds and hence better emulates the lipolytic capability to finish human pancreatic juice. Moreover, porcine pancreatic lipase (PPL) has been appeared to have practically identical stomach-related properties to that of HPL [13].

Human duodenal liquid contains pancreatic lipase and its colipase as the primary lipases and other lipolytic chemicals, for example, carboxylester hydrolase, pancreatic lipase related protein two and phospholipase A, the majority of these catalysts being likewise present in PPE alongside proteases, amylases and contaminations comprising of inorganic and natural material.

Calcium, which is a piece of the inorganic material in PPE, affects the pancreatic lipase activity, in any event *in vitro*. Calcium produces insoluble soaps with the free fatty fats and in this manner, permits the evacuation of FFAs, which will slow down lipolysis from the emulsion surface [14].

PHARMACOKINETIC ASPECTS OF LIPID-BASED FORMULATIONS (LBFS)

The pharmacokinetic aspects of LBFs are shown in Fig. (**1**) and discussed below:

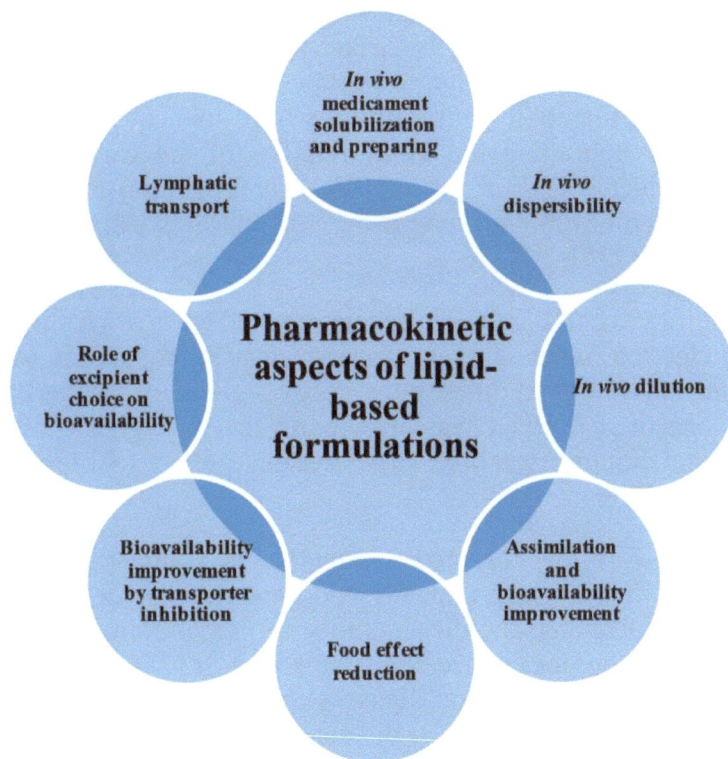

Fig. (1). Various aspects of LBFs regarding Pharmacokinetic.

In Vivo Drug Solubilization and Preparing

Lipids are depicted as crucial ingredients in LBFs; they are primary groups of ingredients in the meal. The digestion of the lipidic ingredients having drugs is basically like that of dietary lipids that are present in a meal. Intake of lipidic preparations brings about an increment in the aggregate of lipids existing in the GI tract. This bigger amount of lipid is best for stimulating the secretion of extra bile *via* contraction of the gallbladder in this manner, expanding luminal concentration of bile salts. The increased intensities of endogenous BS, phospholipids (PLs) and the cholesterol in the occurrence of lipid and surfactants give a lipidic micro-milieu to create globules that will additionally change into different parts such as the vesicular and micellar phases. The drug of BCS II and IV class at first dissolved in the preparation will partition into these. At that point, the drug is partitioned into the generated micelles due to the blend of BS, PLs and cholesterol that is known as "mixed micelles." Their generation is an essential step for solubilization.

The partition of the drug into the lipidic center of micellar systems generates a concentration gradient over the luminal wall that is essential for the retention mechanism. The innate BS behaves as surfactants and helps in the solubilization of the drug by enhancing wettability. This procedure offers an intestinal milieu with an elevated solubilization limit with respect to inadequately water-soluble drugs, subsequently upgrading the bioavailability of the candidate. Different analyses were conducted to find out the drug solubilization in various phases produced amid lipid digestion utilizing combined phase investigations combined with solubility studies [15].

The delivery of drug over the colloidal species created amid *in vivo* digestion was observed with electron paramagnetic resonance spectroscopy. *In vitro* tests, the phases occurring amid luminal digestion, are investigated by adding BS, PLs and cholesterol to intestinal fluid. It was also found that at higher levels of lipids results in different liquid crystalline structures that are available amid *in vivo* digestion.

LCTs are observed to be digested gradually in contrast to MCTs, thus demonstrating that lipase action depends upon the chain length of lipids. This clearly shows that enhancing the dispersibility of preparation by increasing the surfactants concentration does not really enhance the *in vivo* effectiveness of the preparation. The effectiveness of lipases on exposed surface zone was investigated which was also affected by the quantity and size of emulsion droplets that demonstrate the significance of formulation dispersibility [16].

In Vivo Dispersibility and Effect on Pharmacokinetics

Two essential qualities of the LBFs for critical contact with respect to the *in vivo* bioavailability are *in vivo* dispersibility and dilution behavior. The *in vivo* dispersibility can be estimated *in vitro* after diluting preparation into different biorelevant fluids such as FaSSGF, FaSSIF and FeSSIF and estimating the globule size using the dynamic light scattering method.

This would give a reasonable comprehension of *in vivo* dilution performance of the formulation in the stomach and intestinal conditions. All in all, the lesser the globules size, increment in surface area that leads to more lipidic digestion. It has been demonstrated that preparations having smaller globules size will deliver greater bioavailability with lessened individual pharmacokinetic fluctuation. It has been demonstrated that formulations creating smaller globules will deliver greater bioavailability with a decreased inter-subject variation.

It can be reasoned that droplet size isn't a vital marker of the *in vivo* effectiveness and the fate of the inadequately water-soluble drug. This basically relies on the dilution factor and retention, because they decide solubilization or precipitation of the drug. This evidently shows the significance of keeping up drugs in a soluble form for improved retention instead of accelerating the dilution in larger amounts of biological fluids in gastric and intestinal parts [17].

In Vivo Dilution and Effect on Pharmacokinetics

Following dilution in the GI tract, formulation development can give a comprehension about the precipitation of a drug, which is investigated by the optical microscopic examination by *in vitro* dilution in the biological fluids. The equilibrium solubility in an aqueous further to formulations can be considered, which would give a comprehension of the drug precipitation because of water consumption. The quantity of drug precipitation relies upon the formulation parameters and the physiological aspects of the person under drug. While formulation aspects can be controlled, physiological aspects can't be controlled demonstrating the significance of guaranteeing the solubilized form utilizing different *in vitro* tools. The physiologically associated drug precipitation would prompt conflicting pharmacokinetic profiles prompting more significant inter-subject variability [18].

These outcomes demonstrate the significance of the choice of reasonable LBFs for keeping up a drug in solubilized form and furthermore show that the formulation researchers ought to not just think about the physical appearance as an extreme viewpoint about precipitation of inadequately water-soluble drug in the system. While preparing drugs in Type II is by all accounts an alluring decision for avoiding drug precipitation, different perspectives are additionally considered for keeping up the drug in a solubilized form devoid of *in vivo* precipitation. The most intriguing methodology for the development of solubilized drug formation *in vivo* is by joining of hydrophilic polymeric ingredients in the preparation behaves as precipitation inhibitors. This method is extremely helpful for drugs with low solubility in the lipidic ingredients and consequently need a high dose. They can fundamentally postpone precipitation time and if the precipitation time arises more prominent than average retention time, then the degree of retention of an ineffectively water-soluble drug can be enlarged, thereby improving bioavailability. The majority of the regularly utilized polymers in this classification are HPMC, MC, sodium CMC and PVP. The utilization of the polymers as precipitation inhibitors are constrained by LBFs and different formulations such as solid dispersions and controlled release tablet formulations [16]. Yamashita *et al.,* developed utilization of HPMC as precipitation inhibitor for the liberation of tacrolimus as solid dispersions wherein it showed a ten times increment in the AUC and C_{max} when compared with a crystalline powder [19].

Assimilation and Bioavailability Improvement

The essential characteristic by which lipidic formulations upgrade the retention and bioavailability of ineffectively water-soluble drugs is by showing the drug in the soluble state throughout GI tract with negligible precipitation. A variety of mechanisms have been expressed for upgradation of bioavailability such as secretions of pancreatic and biliary juice, extending GI residence time to delay delivery of assimilation and increment in the time accessible for dispersion or dissolution, stimulation of lymphatic transportation, expanding permeability of the intestinal membrane, decreased efflux transporter action by adding ingredients that behave as efflux pump inhibitors and so on as shown in Fig. (**2**). These various mechanisms unmistakably demonstrate the benefits of utilizing LBFs for improving bioavailability. It is likewise clear that regardless of whether a few instruments from the above expressed work for a drug planned in LBFs, it would prompt improved bioavailability along these lines, thus upgrading pharmacological action. The most critical and established case in the bioavailability upgrade by LBFs is Sandimmunes and Sandimmune Neorals formulations of cyclosporine A by Novartis [20, 21].

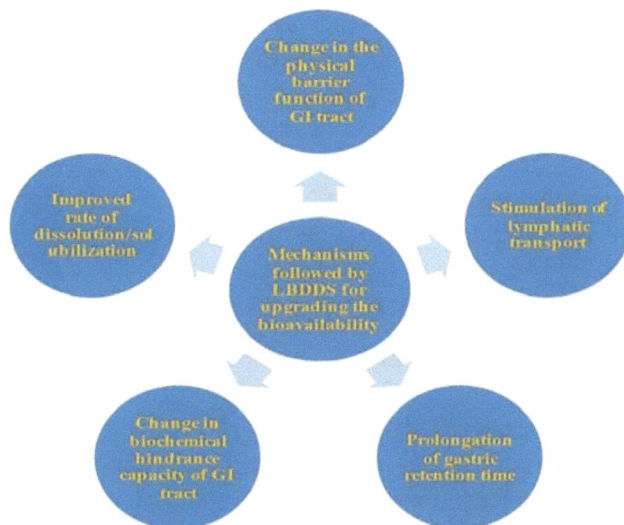

Fig. (2). Mechanisms followed by LBDDS for upgrading the bioavailability.

Role of Selected Ingredient on Bioavailability

There are extensive alternatives of ingredients accessible for formulation inadequately water-soluble drugs in LBFs. The typical ingredients existing in LBFs are lipids, surfactants, hydrophilic solvents and co-solvents.

From a formulation viewpoint, the ingredients selection will affect the drug load, dispersion features, solubilization and stability of drug. Be that as it may, it is likewise essential to judge ingredients from pharmacokinetic viewpoints which can at last influence the bioavailability.

Lymphatic Transport

While lymphatic transportation is specifically corresponding to lipophilicity, a drug particle with a partition coefficient (log P) 4.5 and TG solubility (450 mg/ml) can be compelled to be consumed by means of lymphatic transport utilizing LBFs as opposed through portal vein and liver. Amid lipolysis in the GIT, digestion products like unsaturated fats and MGs are joined with PLs and cholesterol, and enter in enterocyte to formulate TGs. The created TGs entrapped drugs are packed into chylomicrons and in this manner, these enter into the lymphatic system by evading the liver and anticipating hepatic metabolism. This is the primary underlying procedure for lymphatic retention intervened by developing drug with LCT as comparative to MCT and SCT into LBFs. The degree of saturation and quantity of lipids are likewise established to affect the lymphatic transport of drug atoms.

Lymphatic transportation is an alluring assimilation pathway for improving bioavailability of hydrophobic drugs. The favorable mechanism of lymphatic retention is bypassing hepatic metabolism. Among different animal models accessible for investigation of lymphatic transportation of little particles, a model of the rat with a cannulated mesenteric lymph duct is broadly utilized. Different models like sheep and dogs are generally utilized for investigating lymphatic transportation following parental and oral administration respectively [22].

Reduction of Food Effect

Food effect is defined as enhancing or reducing the rate and extent of drug retention in the existence of the meal. It relies upon various factors emerging from physiology, dosage form and physio-chemical characteristics. A variety of aspects, for example, improved solubility within sight of fatty contents of the meal, stimulation of bile secretion, surfactant impacts by meal components and delay in gastric emptying to upgrade the retention time and inhibition of efflux transporters by the composition of a meal are perceived as potential mechanisms for bioavailability upgrade of inadequately soluble drugs with the meal [23].

It has additionally been demonstrated that a couple of lipidic ingredients in the meal can upgrade the chylomicron generation and be able to empower the lymphatic transportation to improve the bioavailability. Thus it is clear that if a suitable combination of lipid and surfactant are selected for developing an inadequately water-soluble drug, they can likewise go about as surrogates for meal segments and thereby invalidating the meal impact and expanding quiet consistency by maintaining a strategic distance from the high-fat dinner utilization with dosage form [24].

The lessening in the meal impact for itraconazole by utilizing SMEDDS preparation was accounted for in healthy volunteers. SMEDDS preparation showed improved C_{max} and AUC esteems under both fasting and feeding states that demonstrated an inconsequential meal impact [25].

Bioavailability Improvement by Transporter Inhibition

These are present in the intestine and recognized to lessen the bioavailability of numerous drugs. BCS class-II won't have the capacity to saturate these such as P-gp present in intestine, subsequently restricting their bioavailability. It was likewise revealed that bioavailability and biological action of numerous anti-neoplastic agents had definitely been diminished because of the activity of drug efflux transporters [26].

CONSENT FOR PUBLICATION

Not applicable.

CONFLICT OF INTEREST

The author declares no conflict of interest, financial or otherwise.

ACKNOWLEDGEMENTS

Declared none.

REFERENCES

[1]   Xiao L, Yi T, Liu Y, Zhou H. The *in vitro* lipolysis of lipid-based drug delivery systems: A newly identified relationship between drug release and liquid crystalline phase. BioMed Res Int 2016; 2016(8)2364317
[PMID: 27294110]

[2]   Guyer RA, Macara IG. Loss of the polarity protein PAR3 activates STAT3 signaling *via* an atypical protein kinase C (aPKC)/NF-κB/interleukin-6 (IL-6) axis in mouse mammary cells. J Biol Chem 2015; 290(13): 8457-68.
[http://dx.doi.org/10.1074/jbc.M114.621011] [PMID: 25657002]

[3]   Dahan A, Hoffman A. Rationalizing the selection of oral lipid based drug delivery systems by an *in vitro* dynamic lipolysis model for improved oral bioavailability of poorly water soluble drugs. J Control Release 2008; 129(1): 1-10.
[http://dx.doi.org/10.1016/j.jconrel.2008.03.021] [PMID: 18499294]

[4]   Mercuri A, Curto AL, Wickham MSJ, Barker SA. Dynamic gastric model (DGM): A novel *in vitro* apparatus to assess the impact of gastric digestion on the droplet size of self-emulsifying drug-delivery systems. J Pharma Pharmacol 2008; 3(96): 33-47.

[5]   Porter CJ, Pouton CW, Cuine JF, Charman WN. Enhancing intestinal drug solubilisation using lipid-based delivery systems. Adv Drug Deliv Rev 2008; 60(6): 673-91.
[http://dx.doi.org/10.1016/j.addr.2007.10.014] [PMID: 18155801]

[6]   Larsen AT, Sassene P, Müllertz A. *In vitro* lipolysis models as a tool for the characterization of oral lipid and surfactant based drug delivery systems. Int J Pharm 2011; 417(1-2): 245-55.
[http://dx.doi.org/10.1016/j.ijpharm.2011.03.002] [PMID: 21392564]

[7]   Vithani K, Hawley A, Jannin V, Pouton C, Boyd BJ. Inclusion of digestible surfactants in solid SMEDDS formulation removes lag time and influences the formation of structured particles during digestion. AAPS J 2017; 19(3): 754-64.
[http://dx.doi.org/10.1208/s12248-016-0036-6] [PMID: 28116678]

[8]   Mun S, Decker EA, McClements DJ. Influence of emulsifier type on *in vitro* digestibility of lipid droplets by pancreatic lipase. Food Res Int 2007; 40(6): 770-81.
[http://dx.doi.org/10.1016/j.foodres.2007.01.007]

[9]   Dahan A, Hoffman A. The effect of different lipid based formulations on the oral absorption of lipophilic drugs: the ability of *in vitro* lipolysis and consecutive *ex vivo* intestinal permeability data to predict *in vivo* bioavailability in rats. Eur J Pharm Biopharm 2007; 67(1): 96-105.
[http://dx.doi.org/10.1016/j.ejpb.2007.01.017] [PMID: 17329087]

[10]   Zangenberg NH, Müllertz A, Kristensen HG, Hovgaard L. A dynamic in vitro lipolysis model. I. Controlling the rate of lipolysis by continuous addition of calcium. Eur J Pharm Sci 2001; 14(2): 115-22.

[http://dx.doi.org/10.1016/S0928-0987(01)00169-5] [PMID: 11500257]

[11]   Larsen AT, Ohlsson AG, Polentarutti B, *et al.* Oral bioavailability of cinnarizine in dogs: relation to SNEDDS droplet size, drug solubility and *in vitro* precipitation. Eur J Pharm Sci 2013; 48(1-2): 339-50.
[http://dx.doi.org/10.1016/j.ejps.2012.11.004] [PMID: 23178440]

[12]   Williams HD, Anby MU, Sassene P, *et al.* Toward the establishment of standardized *in vitro* tests for lipid-based formulations. 2. The effect of bile salt concentration and drug loading on the performance of type I, II, IIIA, IIIB, and IV formulations during *in vitro* digestion. Mol Pharm 2012; 9(11): 3286-300.
[http://dx.doi.org/10.1021/mp300331z] [PMID: 23030411]

[13]   Griffin BT, Kuentz M, Vertzoni M, *et al.* Comparison of *in vitro* tests at various levels of complexity for the prediction of *in vivo* performance of lipid-based formulations: case studies with fenofibrate. Eur J Pharm Biopharm 2014; 86(3): 427-37.
[http://dx.doi.org/10.1016/j.ejpb.2013.10.016] [PMID: 24184675]

[14]   Sassene P, Kleberg K, Williams HD, *et al.* Toward the establishment of standardized *in vitro* tests for lipid-based formulations, part 6: effects of varying pancreatin and calcium levels. AAPS J 2014; 16(6): 1344-57.
[http://dx.doi.org/10.1208/s12248-014-9672-x] [PMID: 25274609]

[15]   Kossena GA, Charman WN, Boyd BJ, Dunstan DE, Porter CJ. Probing drug solubilization patterns in the gastrointestinal tract after administration of lipid-based delivery systems: a phase diagram approach. J Pharm Sci 2004; 93(2): 332-48.
[http://dx.doi.org/10.1002/jps.10554] [PMID: 14705191]

[16]   Sek L, Porter CJ, Kaukonen AM, Charman WN. Evaluation of the in-vitro digestion profiles of long and medium chain glycerides and the phase behaviour of their lipolytic products. J Pharm Pharmacol 2002; 54(1): 29-41.
[http://dx.doi.org/10.1211/0022357021771896] [PMID: 11833493]

[17]   Trull AK, Tan KK, Tan L, Alexander GJ, Jamieson NV. Absorption of cyclosporin from conventional and new microemulsion oral formulations in liver transplant recipients with external biliary diversion. Br J Clin Pharmacol 1995; 39(6): 627-31.
[http://dx.doi.org/10.1111/j.1365-2125.1995.tb05722.x] [PMID: 7654480]

[18]   Narang AS, Delmarre D, Gao D. Stable drug encapsulation in micelles and microemulsions. Int J Pharm 2007; 345(1-2): 9-25.
[http://dx.doi.org/10.1016/j.ijpharm.2007.08.057] [PMID: 17945446]

[19]   Yamashita K, Nakate T, Okimoto K, *et al.* Establishment of new preparation method for solid dispersion formulation of tacrolimus. Int J Pharm 2003; 267(1-2): 79-91.
[http://dx.doi.org/10.1016/j.ijpharm.2003.07.010] [PMID: 14602386]

[20]   Porter CJ, Trevaskis NL, Charman WN. Lipids and lipid-based formulations: optimizing the oral delivery of lipophilic drugs. Nat Rev Drug Discov 2007; 6(3): 231-48.
[http://dx.doi.org/10.1038/nrd2197] [PMID: 17330072]

[21]   Gao ZG, Choi HG, Shin HJ, *et al.* Physicochemical characterization and evaluation of a microemulsion system for oral delivery of cyclosporin A. Int J Pharm 1998; 161(1): 75-86.
[http://dx.doi.org/10.1016/S0378-5173(97)00325-6]

[22]   Caliph SM, Charman WN, Porter CJ. Effect of short-, medium-, and long-chain fatty acid-based vehicles on the absolute oral bioavailability and intestinal lymphatic transport of halofantrine and assessment of mass balance in lymph-cannulated and non-cannulated rats. J Pharm Sci 2000; 89(8): 1073-84.
[http://dx.doi.org/10.1002/1520-6017(200008)89:8<1073::AID-JPS12>3.0.CO;2-V]   [PMID: 10906731]

[23]   Custodio JM, Wu CY, Benet LZ. Predicting drug disposition, absorption/elimination/transporter

interplay and the role of food on drug absorption. Adv Drug Deliv Rev 2008; 60(6): 717-33.
[http://dx.doi.org/10.1016/j.addr.2007.08.043] [PMID: 18199522]

[24] Hauss DJ. Oral lipid-based formulations. Adv Drug Deliv Rev 2007; 59(7): 667-76.
[http://dx.doi.org/10.1016/j.addr.2007.05.006] [PMID: 17618704]

[25] Woo JS, Song YK, Hong JY, Lim SJ, Kim CK. Reduced food-effect and enhanced bioavailability of a self-microemulsifying formulation of itraconazole in healthy volunteers. Eur J Pharm Sci 2008; 33(2): 159-65.
[http://dx.doi.org/10.1016/j.ejps.2007.11.001] [PMID: 18178070]

[26] Gottesman MM, Fojo T, Bates SE. Multidrug resistance in cancer: role of ATP-dependent transporters. Nat Rev Cancer 2002; 2(1): 48-58.
[http://dx.doi.org/10.1038/nrc706] [PMID: 11902585]

SUBJECT INDEX

A

Absorption 30, 31, 46, 47, 50, 65, 74, 147
  cellular 74
  oral 37, 46
  pathway 50
Absorptive cells 50, 123, 170
  fundamental intestinal 50
Acesulfame potassium 123
Acid 19, 21, 24, 34, 41, 50, 68, 69, 88, 90, 96,
     98, 101, 104, 107, 118, 138, 160, 161,
     162, 164, 173, 174, 175, 177, 178
  Acetylsalicylic 118
  ascorbic 19, 24, 68, 69
  azelaic 68
  caprylic capric 160
  formulated betulinic 19
  free fatty (FFAs) 175, 177, 178
  hyaluronic 104
  long-chain fatty (LCFA) 96, 107, 173, 177
  oleanic 164
  oleic 90, 138, 161, 162, 177
  ricinoleic 88
  salicylic 41, 50, 69, 98
  sorbic 21
  stearic 101
  succinic 19
  tetra-acidic 174
  valproic 34
Acidic 118, 176
  chyme 176
  milieu 118
Action 121, 181
  decreased efflux transporter 181
  thermodynamic 121
Activity 34, 106, 175, 183
  lymphotropic 106
Acute 105, 123
  pro-myelocytic leukemia 123
  respiratory syndrome-related coronavirus
    105
Adhesion 40

Amorphous solid dispersion (ASD) 144
Amphiphilic copolymers 10
Ampholytic surfactants 87
Anionic carrier encoun-ters electrostatic
    repulsion 100
Antineoplastic agents 99, 105
Antioxidants 90, 91, 92, 157
  lipid-soluble 91
Artemisia argyi oil (AAO) 36
Assimilation 64, 72, 100, 173, 174
  dissolution-rate-limited 64
  interface amid 174
  liposomal 100
  medicaments 72
  phospholipids amid 173
Atractylodes extract 10

B

Bile 44, 47, 48, 49, 106, 108, 119, 169, 172,
    173, 174, 175, 177, 179, 183
  salts (BS) 44, 47, 48, 49, 106, 108, 119,
    169, 172, 173, 174, 175, 177, 179
  secretion 183
Biliary 51, 181
  juice 181
  lipids 51
Bioseparations by microemulsions 59, 71
Blood 2, 5, 49, 50, 67, 85, 96, 97, 98, 99, 101,
    103, 104, 105, 146, 169
  capillary endothelium 49
  circulation 5, 85, 96, 99, 105, 146
  plasma exposure 103
  systematic 49, 50
  systemic 49, 103
Bragg's law 71

C

Calcium 173, 174, 175, 176, 177, 178
  bioavailability 176
  chelation 174

www.ingramcontent.com/pod-product-compliance
Lightning Source LLC
Chambersburg PA
CBHW050846220326

41598CB00006B/443